The Chinese Herbal Cookbook

Healing Foods for Inner Balance

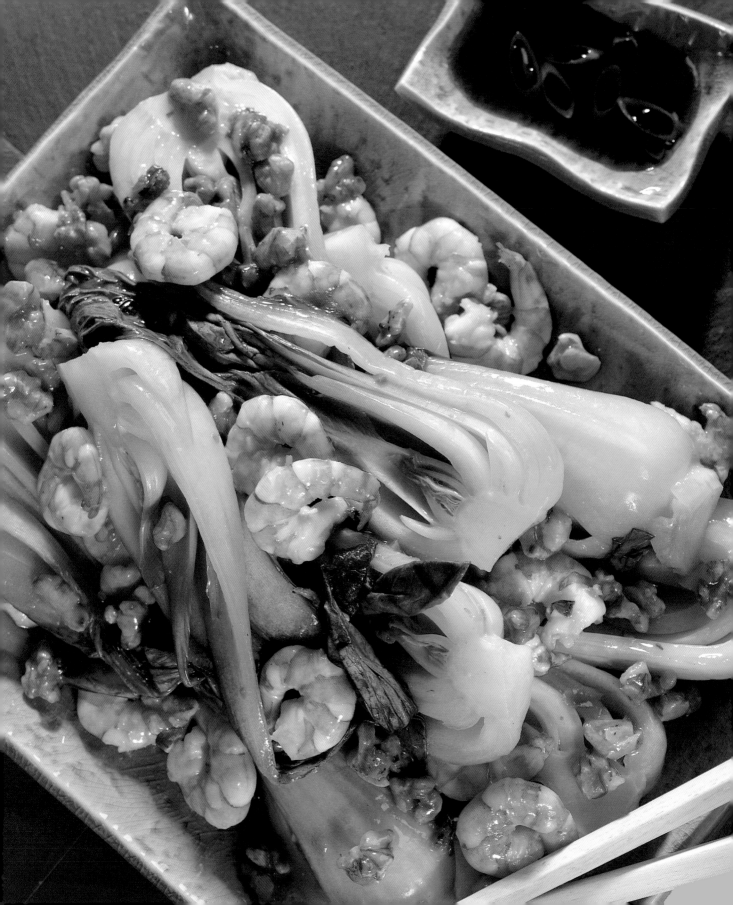

The Chinese Herbal Cookbook

Healing Foods for Inner Balance

Penelope Ody

with Alice Lyon and Dragana Vilinac

Weatherhill

First edition, 2001

© 2000 by Penelope Ody, Alice Lyon & Dragana Vilinac

Edited by Caroline Taggart
Copy-edited by Anne Sheasby
Designed by Peter Butler
Photography by Julie Dixon
Home economy by Kathy Man
Calligraphy by Xing Liu
Production by Lorraine Baird and Sha Huxtable
Printed in Singapore by Kyodo Printing Co.

ISBN 0-8348-0480-8
Library of Congress Cataloging in Publication data available.

Authors' acknowledgements
The authors would like to thank Robert Miller, Margot Nielsen, Lei Zhou An, Julia Jus, and Charlotte Lyon for sharing their ideas and offering helpful comments and suggestions.

The publishers would like to thank W. Wing Lip plc for generously supplying utensils for photography and Thomas Goode, David Mellor, Neal Street East and The Pier for the loan of china and other props

**Previous page: Shrimp and walnut stir-fry
(recipe on page 152)**

Contents

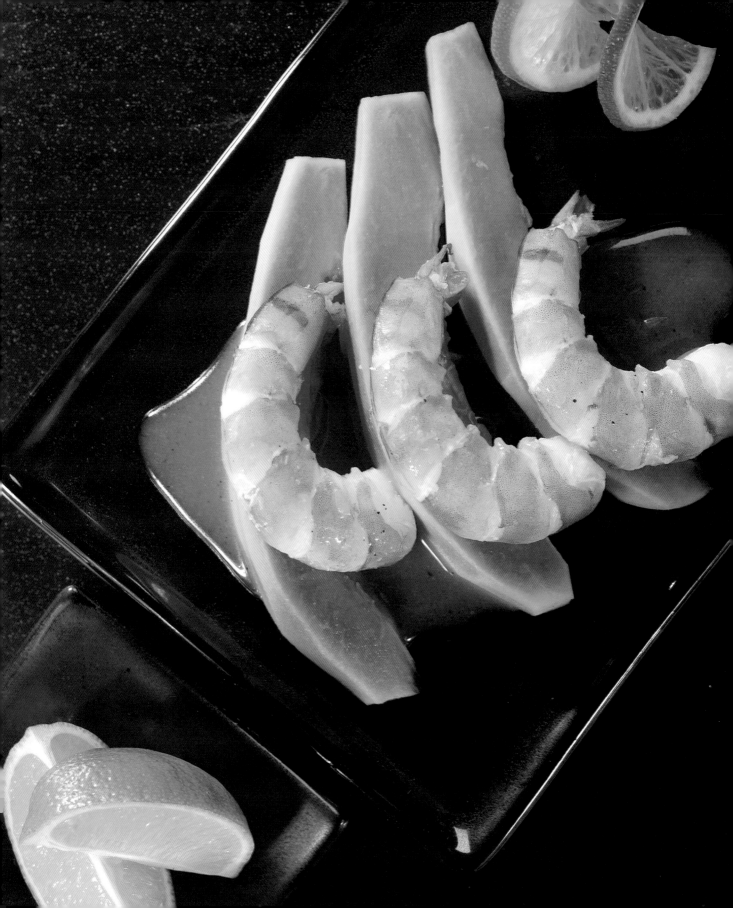

Introduction

Healthy eating has become one of the preoccupations of our age. Over the past few years, our concerns have ranged from the need to avoid high cholesterol foods to worries about genetically modified produce. Intensive farming practices have alerted us all to the risk of poor animal hygiene and welfare as successive food scares have made *Salmonella, Listeria, E. coli* or BSE depressingly familiar. We worry about pesticides in our apples, growth hormones in our beef and "Round-Up resistance" in our soya. We also take supplements of vitamins and minerals to replace those essential nutrients which can no longer be guaranteed in the highly processed, over-pre-served ingredients on supermarket shelves.

But these preoccupations completely neglect something which our ancestors took for granted: the need to balance the character of various foods to avoid any detrimental side-effects they may have and the ability to use the therapeutic properties of those same foods to improve and preserve health.

Certainly, we know that broccoli is rich in ACE vitamins, which are important in anti-cancer diets. We may even eat high-zinc foods, such as pumpkin seeds, to help strengthen the immune system. But we also think nothing of eating strawberries or cucumbers in the depth of winter – something our ancestors would have dismissed as a sure way to encourage stomach chills and watery diarrhoea as these intrinsically "cold" foods combine with the cold climate, to attack our vital inner heat.

At the same time, the range and availability of fresh herbs continues to expand. Today, we can buy lemon grass or ginger in supermarkets, fresh shiitake mushrooms are readily available and pots of young basil plants can be found throughout the year. Many cooks happily use these fashionable ingredients but few will be aware that they are adding rather more than flavour to their dishes. These herbs, mushrooms, fruits and vegetables – along with meats and fish – are more than pleasant nutrients, they can have a very real effect on our physiology and well-being. They're also a much more pleasurable way to stay healthy than dosing with patent medicines, pharmaceutical drugs or a growing assortment of nutritional supplements.

The recipes in this book not only reflect our training as medical herbalists in European and Chinese traditions, but also bring a cross-section of cooking styles and tastes which echo our own lifestyles as working women or a mother of small children, juggling family and professional demands in town or country, East or West.

Many of the dishes are very quick and easy to prepare – ideal when time and energies are in short supply at the end of a busy working day. Others are more leisurely and occasionally a little complex. However, while we're all enthusiastic amateur cooks, our training is in medical rather than culinary skills – none of the dishes demands "cordon bleu" abilities and while some are clearly for special occasions and grander meals, most are ideal for the informal family lunches and suppers we all normally cook.

PENELOPE ODY

Prawns and papaya (recipe on page 100)

Chinese Medicine and Food

Over the past two decades, traditional Chinese medicine, once regarded as an obscure and exotic study, has become commonplace in the West. Over-the-counter medicines based on ancient formulae are now readily available from many pharmacists and health food shops, while *Dang Gui* (Chinese angelica) has joined ginseng as one of the West's favourite tonic remedies.

But Chinese medicine is much more than acupuncture and Western-style pills or capsules. Like Ayurvedic medicine in India, it is a way of life: a combination of regular exercises, familiar in the West as *t'ai-chi* or *Qigong*, meals based on traditional health-giving recipes and an emphasis on maintaining harmony with the natural environment that goes back to the ancient Taoists.

The theories that still guide Chinese practitioners date to 2500 B.C. when Shen Nong, the "divine farmer" taught mankind how to cultivate grains and reputedly tasted hundreds of herbs to identify their healing properties. As in Europe in those far-off times, medicine, religion and philosophy were closely intertwined and the Taoists linked prosperity, longevity and health with following the way of "virtue". Virtue meant conforming to nature and living in harmony with all things and this close association with the natural world can still be seen in the five-element model and the theory of *yin* and *yang,* which form the basis of traditional Chinese medicine (TCM).

A Pattern of Fives

Living close to nature, those early Chinese thinkers were acutely aware of the changing seasons and saw a pattern of five basic elements in the world around them. Heavy winter rains caused new plants to emerge in the spring; these in turn were scorched during the summer heat, leading to forest fires which created ashes to be returned to earth, already known as the source of valuable metal ores. Metal surfaces conducted heat and so tended to be cold, thus causing water to condense – and start the cycle once more, with winter rains encouraging the plants to grow.

These simple observations developed into what is now known as the five-phase or five-element model (see diagram) linking Water, Wood, Fire, Earth and Metal. Water promotes or gives rise to Wood, which promotes Fire, which in turn gives rise to Earth, which promotes Metal, which leads back to Water. But the orderly Chinese mind did not limit this model to simple elements. Since all things in nature were one, then all things in nature must also conform to this model and so a complex series of fives began to be associated with the five elements: five seasons, five directions, five colours, five solid body organs, five emotions, five tastes, five sounds, five smells – and so on.

The five basic elements interact to control and regulate each other so any imbalance in one element affects the whole cycle. Too much Water and Fire becomes weak, if Metal is weak then Wood gets out of hand. This interaction also applies to the bodily organs which are associated with each of the elements. "Over-exuberant liver" (Wood) affects the spleen/stomach (Earth) so upsets digestion, for example.

The five-element model also includes tastes which are believed to have a specific impact on the particular organs, fluids and emotions associated with them.

Tasty Options

The five classic tastes of pungent, sweet, sour, bitter and salty each has its own particular effect on the body and, like the seasons, the taste of food can similarly affect the five element cycle with excess or shortages leading to imbalance. Certain tastes may need to be avoided if the associated organ is weak – excessive sweet tastes, for example, can affect some digestive disorders, while salty tastes will increase oedema and water retention because of their affect on the kidney.

A good balance of tastes is important to maintain health and any diet which allows one to become over-dominant – such as the Western fondness for sweet tastes from unrefined sugars and avoidance of highly flavoured, pungent dishes, can lead to illness. Health is maintained by the right balance of tastes while disharmonies can be corrected by adjusting the flavour of particular meals.

The five classic tastes are sometimes augmented with the addition of two further categories – astringent and bland/neutral – to cover the full range of herbal and food options. This intrinsic character of foods and herbs is indicated in the recipes.

The sour flavour enters into the liver; the pungent flavour enters into the lungs; the bitter flavour enters into the heart; the salty flavour enters into the kidneys; and the sweet flavour enters into the spleen… The pungent flavour goes into the respiratory tract; when there is illness in the respiratory tract one should not eat too much pungent food. The salty flavour goes into the blood; when there is disease in the blood one should not eat too much salty food. The bitter flavour goes into the bones; when there is a disease of the bones one should not eat too much bitter food.

HUANG DI: *YELLOW EMPEROR'S CANON OF INTERNAL MEDICINE*
(C. 2500 BC)

Yin and *Yang*

To the five-element model, the Taoists added two great forces – *yin* and *yang* – as alternating aspects of the creative force central to all things. These two opposites could be seen as the light and dark sides of the mountain, the above and below, the outside and inside – paired, inseparable and vital.

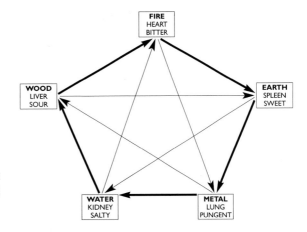

Yang is sometimes described in the West as the more "masculine" aspect – movement, strength, outgoing, active – while *yin* is couched in traditional feminine terms: static, frailty, inward-looking, passive. It is a rather artificial approach as *yin* and *yang* are equal and contained in all

Five-Element Associations

	Wood	**Fire**	**Earth**	**Metal**	**Water**
Direction	East	South	Centre	West	North
Colour	Green	Red	Yellow	White	Black
Season	Spring	Summer	Late Summer (traditionally from c. July 7 for a month)	Autumn	Winter
Climate	Wind	Hot	Dampness	Dryness	Cold
Solid organ (*Zang*)	Liver	Heart	Spleen	Lung	Kidney
Hollow organ (*Fu*)	Gall bladder	Small Intestine	Stomach	Large Intestine	Urinary Bladder
Sense organs/openings	Eyes Sight	Tongue Speech	Mouth Taste	Nose Smell	Ears Hearing
Emotion	Anger	Joy/Fright	Worry	Sadness/Grief	Fear
Taste	Sour	Bitter	Sweet	Pungent/Acrid	Salty
Tissues	Tendon Nails	Blood vessels Complexion	Muscles Lips	Skin Body hair	Bone Head hair
Sound	Shouting	Laughing	Singing	Weeping	Groaning
Smell	Rancid	Burnt	Fragrant	Rotten	Putrid
Body fluid	Tears	Sweat	Saliva	Mucus	Urine
Meat	Chicken	Mutton	Beef	Horse	Pork
Cereal	Wheat	Glutinous millet	Millet	Rice	Beans

things. Both aspects are present at all times: while summer is more strongly *yang*, because it is a hot, bright season it still contains some *yin*; similarly, damp and cold winter is more closely aligned with *yin*, although it still contains a remnant of *yang*.

Foods, too, are affected by this intrinsic balance of *yin* and *yang*. Some are colder and damper – *yin; others are* more heating and dry – *yang.* Just as maintaining the right balance in tastes is important for health, so is the correct mixture of *yin* and *yang* dishes. The "nature" of various foods and herbs is indicated in the recipes.

In ill health, a "cold" condition such as a chill or watery diarrhoea would be treated with warming remedies and foods, while a "hot" problem such as an inflammation, would be treated with cooling remedies.

Healthy people have their own individual bias in basic constitution. Some tend to be more *yin* while others are predominantly *yang*: some tend to feel the cold more, others tend to be hotter and "dry" so may

The Tastes of Some Common Foods
NB: Some foods have more than one flavour

Pungent foods: chives, fennel, garlic, kumquat, leeks, red and green peppers, pepper, rice bran, soybean oil, spring onions, sweet basil, ginger, wine.

Sweet foods: aduki beans, aubergines, bamboo shoots, bean curd, beef, beetroot, broad beans, butter, button mushrooms, calves' liver, carrots, celery, cherries, coffee, chicken, chicken livers, Chinese leaves, cow's milk, cucumber, hen's eggs, honey, lamb's kidney, lamb's liver, lettuce, *Mu Erh* mushrooms, mung beans, peanuts, pork, pumpkins, ripe fruits (including apples, bananas, dates, grapes, oranges, pineapple), shiitake mushrooms, shrimps, sugar, sweet potatoes, wheat, wine.

Sour foods: aduki beans, duck, lemons, mangoes, olives, tomatoes, unripe fruits (such as apples, pears, grapefruit, plums), vinegar.

Bitter foods: asparagus, coffee, hops, lamb's liver, lettuce, pumpkins, vinegar, wine.

Salty foods: barley, chive seeds, clams, crab, duck, ham, oysters, pig's kidney, pork.

Astringent foods: vinegar

Bland/neutral foods: Chinese white fungus

Yin foods are cooler while yang foods are more heating

Cold foods: bamboo shoots, bananas, clams, crab, grapefruit, lettuce, persimmons, seaweed, water chestnuts, watercress, watermelons.

Cool foods: apples, bean curd, button mushrooms, cucumber, lettuce, mangoes, mung beans, pears, spinach, strawberries, tomatoes.

Neutral foods: apricots, beef, beetroot, Chinese leaves, carrots, celery, corn (maize), eggs, honey, polished white rice, potatoes, pumpkins, white sugar.

Warm foods: brown sugar, cherries, chicken, chives, dates, spring onions, ham, kumquats, leeks, mutton, peaches, raspberries, prawns, walnuts, wine, sunflower seeds.

Hot foods: ginger, pepper, green and red peppers, soya bean oil.

always feel thirsty. A hot person should eat more cold foods than average to help maintain an ideal *yin-yang* balance, while someone who is always cold should opt for more warming dishes. Eat a little more of the foods which will help combat any intrinsic imbalances and avoid those which will emphasise such weaknesses.

All Sorts of Directions
Just as foods and herbs are hot or cold, dry or damp, Chinese theory also believes they have a directional effect on energy flows *(Qi)* within the body. They may be described as rising, falling, or moving inwards or outwards. Solid, heavy foods (such as roots) will fall or sink, while lighter foods (such as leaves) will encourage energy to rise or float. Foods which encourage energy flows outwards may increase perspiration and have a cooling effect in fevers, while foods which encourage inward movement may be appropriate in diarrhoea.

In general, meals need to contain a balance of these various types of foods to ensure that the overall effect is neutral. Occasionally, a specific direction may be needed: sufferers from coughs or nausea associated with what the Chinese term rising or rebellious *Qi,* may welcome foods which encourage the energy flows downwards. Those suffering from chronic constipation will welcome foods which move outwards, while frequent urination may be countered by eating foods which encourage inward motion. Foods that are upwards and outwards are better in spring and summer, those that are inwards and downwards are better in autumn and winter.

Organs and Energy

The basic philosophical ideas of five elements and *yin-yang* balance have developed over the last 3000 years into a highly formalised medical theory used to explain illness and bodily functions. The five solid or *Zang* organs (heart, liver, spleen, kidney and lungs), which are *yin* in character, are paired with five *yang* organs or "bowels" — also called hollow or *Fu* organs (small intestine, gall bladder, stomach, urinary bladder and large intestine) — and are connected to them by meridians or acupuncture channels.

When this Chinese model of the human body was first mooted, there were, obviously, no microscopes and no means of studying physiology and detailed anatomy. There was also no separation of the individual into physical, emotional and spiritual entities, so the organs were credited with functions which in Western terms can sound confusing and at times incomprehensible. The liver, for example, is said to "store the soul", while the spleen is responsible for "intention" or "determination" and the kidneys control the process of respiration.

The organs also have many familiar Western attributes and the terms easily become confusing — "stagnating liver *Qi*", for example, would have a range of symptoms associated with emotional upsets and irritability far beyond the anatomical concept of poor liver function.

Encouraging Energy Flows/Directional Foods

Rising/upward foods: aduki beans, apricots, beans, beetroot, black fungus, Chinese leaves, carrots, celery, cow's milk,, duck, figs, grapes, hen's eggs, honey, hyacinth beans, kidney beans, olives, pineapple, pork, potatoes, shiitake mushrooms, sweet potato, white sugar.

Falling/downward foods: apples, aubergines, bamboo shoots, bananas, bean curd, button mushrooms, grapefruit, kumquats, Job's tears, lettuce, mangoes, mung beans, peaches, spinach, strawberries, tangerines, water chestnuts, wheat.

Outward foods: black pepper, ginger, green and red pepper, soya bean oil.

Inward foods: crab, lettuce, seaweeds.

While appropriate foods and herbs can be used to restore the sort of physical imbalance in the organs familiar in the West, these extended Chinese attributes can be treated in the same way. The heart, for example, is associated with the spirit and appropriate behaviour, so a heart herb such as *Fu Ling* (Indian bread), which can be used as a diuretic for heart weaknesses associated with dropsy and fluid retention, is also regarded as a sedative to "calm the spirit" in those suffering from nervous over-excitability or erratic behaviour patterns.

The *Zang* and *Fu* organs are part of a complex network which also involves five fundamental substances. The most familiar of these in the West is *Qi* which is sometimes written as *ch'i* and is usually translated as "vital energy". Its main characteristic is motion — the activity of life. There are very many subdivisions of *Qi*. Some scholars suggest that as many as 32 varieties have been described in Chinese texts over the past 2500 years, as physicians have tried to refine the definitions of these subtle energies.

Basically *Qi* is a mixture of energies derived from the food we eat and the air we breathe, plus an element inherited from our parents which is with us from birth. These raw ingredients then combine and are transformed in a variety of ways to make the different sorts of *Qi* which circulate in the body. *Qi* is also seen as actual activity: the physiological function of the various body organs. Heart *Qi*, for example, is the action of the heart, not just an immaterial sort of energy state.

One type of *Qi* often referred to in the West is *Wei Qi* or "defence energy". This is sometimes equated with our immune system and herbs which stimulate *Wei Qi* are often shown by modern research studies to strengthen the immune system. These herbs become important in *Fu Zheng* therapy (see page 125) and can be used in strengthening dishes to help us combat recurrent infections and other stresses. Another type of *Qi* is *Gu Qi* or "grain *Qi*", produced from food by the spleen, which is then used to make other important sorts of *Qi* used in the body to maintain bodily functions such as respiration or blood circulation.

The other fundamental substances are *Jing* or "essence", *Xue* or "blood", *Jin-Ye* or "body fluids" and *Shen* or "spirit". *Jing* is fundamental to life and essential for reproduction; its gradual decay during our lifetimes is blamed for the range of menopausal symptoms women often experience at the end of their childbearing years. *Jing* is also believed to produce bone marrow, which

Chinese medicine also associates with the brain (described as the "sea of the marrow"), so it is not really surprising that *Jing* tends to be associated with innate creativity. Foods and herbs which encourage *Jing* can be especially helpful in middle age or for those in highly demanding and creative jobs who often become ill as result of the excessive demands they place on *Jing*.

Xue is a rather more tangible entity than *Qi* or *Jing*. It is the familiar red stuff that transports nutrients throughout the body. It is also regarded as essential for mental activities and clear thinking and is closely associated with the liver (which stores blood) and the menstrual cycle. Herbs and foods which nourish blood are among the most important tonic remedies for women.

Jin-Ye is the label used to describe just about any internal liquid or secretion including saliva, gastric juices, phlegm, tears, mucus and sweat. Body fluids are seen as being derived from our food and water and are converted in the spleen and stomach into the *Jin* (clear fluid) and *Ye* (turbid or thick fluid) which nourish the inner parts of the body such as joints, body orifices, brain and bone marrow.

Shen – an even more nebulous concept than *Jing* or *Qi* – is generally translated as "spirit", the inner strength behind both essence and energy, closely associated with human consciousness. It is sometimes described as "awareness" and is linked to lifestyle and creativity. *Jing*, *Qi* and *Shen* are referred to in Chinese tradition as "the three treasures".

Herbs and foods are used to help strengthen these vital fundamental substances to maintain health, so any excesses or deficiencies in the diet in terms of taste, *yin* or *yang* are likely to lead to imbalance and thus ill health.

Rediscovering the Western Diet

"In winter eat as much as possible and drink as little as possible; drink should be wine as undiluted as possible and food should be bread with all meats roasted; during this season take as few vegetables as possible for so will the body be mostly hot and dry…"

HIPPOCRATES *REGIMEN IN HEALTH* (C. 420 BC)

Traditional Chinese theories may seem very strange today in the West, where a "balanced meal" is thought of in terms of the right amount of protein or carbohydrates with a suitable sprinkling of essential minerals or vitamins, but 2500 years ago a "balanced" diet meant something rather more similar to the Chinese concept of the right mix of *yin* and *yang* foods. Around 420 BC, Hippocrates – the Greek physician regarded as the father of modern medicine, who lived and practised on the island of Cos – set out the prevailing theories as a *Regimen in Health* which was to be regarded as a key guide to healthy living for the next two millennia.

Just as in Taoist theories of *yin* and *yang*, he urged matching diet to the changing seasons to ensure that the body was well equipped to combat any prevailing ills. Winter, in much of Europe, was cold and damp so – following the basic tenets of what we now call Galenic Medicine, after the second-century physician who classifed them – it was important to make the body hot and dry to balance out these prevailing characteristics.

Just as in China, this idea of balancing hot and cold, dry and damp, goes back to the early views of the world as composed of basic elements, only in ancient Greek philosophy there are four – Fire, Earth, Water and Air – rather than five (see diagram). These not only formed the world around us, but also controlled the physical and emotional aspects of every man and

Classification of Some Herbs and Foods According to Hippocrates

Cool: lettuce, purslane (fresh), endive.

Hot: garlic, onions, cress, mustard, rocket, mint, sorrel, cabbage, pennyroyal, marjoram, savory, almonds, purslane (dried), blite (spinach), lentils.

Damp: red orach (a salad herb).

Dry: rue, asparagus, sage, millet.

Damp and hot: leeks, pumpkins, turnips, mulberries, pears, grapes, green figs, radishes.

Damp and cold: oats, barley.

Dry and hot: honey, coriander, anise, basil, hyssop, thyme.

woman and influenced the "humours" which were a product of digestion and affected health and well-being. Too much heat and dryness and yellow bile or the "choleric" humour would become dominant, leading to bad temper, irritability and inflammations. Too much cold and damp and there would be a surfeit of "phlegm", leaving the sufferer lethargic, lacking in energy and probably with nasal congestion or muscular aches. Other imbalances resulted in an excess of "black bile" or "melancholic humour" or blood (sanguine humour).

Diet could be used to combat the effects of the changing seasons and maintain balance. So, Hippocrates urged that in spring as the temperature increased, we should eat boiled meats instead of roasted, along with raw or boiled vegetables and plenty of well-diluted drinks. In the heat of summer, those drinks should be "diluted and copious", as the season was "hot and dry and makes bodies burning and parched": small meals and minimal meat were the order of the day. As the damp autumn arrived, he advised "abundant and drier" meals and fewer drinks "for in this way a man will be most healthy and least chilly as the season is cold and wet".

Autumn and winter are times for strengthening and fortifying foods to combat the cold, dark, damp days: plenty of sweet tastes, "hot" meats and root vegetables. Spring and summer, in contrast, need light, moister dishes to encourage elimination and clear the body of heat and toxic wastes: plenty of bitter flavours, salads and fish. Traditional European eating habits often reflect these patterns; Christmas lunch with its roast meat and plum pudding is ideal for the shortest days of the year, while the abstinence once commonplace in Lent provided a good cleansing spring treatment. The seasonal patterns of berry fruits in summer and game in autumn are just as appropriate.

These same ideas were still prevalent in Elizabethan England when the great herbalist John Gerard warned against eating strawberries in cold weather or on a "cold stomicke" as this would increase the "phlegmatic humours" and lead to digestive upsets. Instead, he recommended them to "quench thirst, cooleth heate of the stomicke and inflammation of the liver".

Just as in Chinese theory individuals tend to be predominantly *yin* or *yang*, so in Galenic theory they had their dominant humour with people described as having a "choleric" or "sanguine" disposition. Food could be used to adjust these imbalances in order to create the harmonious ideal where no humour was especially dominant.

While each food had its dominant characteristics and

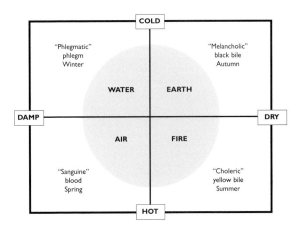

could be used in illness or imbalance, to restore order, in health the overall effect of the meal should be neutral: it should be adjusted by matching hot or dry substances with cold or damp ones. This wasn't an activity confined to skilled chefs or physicians, but was an established style of cooking which most housewives followed, although the underlying theory was gradually forgotten. As the English physician and herbalist Nicholas Culpeper put it in 1653: "One good old fashion is not yet left off, viz. to boil fennel with fish: for it consumes that phlegmatic humour which fish most plentifully afford and annoy the body with, though few that use it know wherefore they do it."

As in China, herbs and foods were classified in terms of their dominant character – cold, hot, dry or damp. Meat tended to be heating and the cooking method (as Hippocrates points out) could make it hotter still; fish was damp; fresh beans and apples were cold and moist; wheat was generally hot and moist, and so on. Food intake, like the prevailing seasons, was considered to have a direct action on the four humours – blood, phlegm, yellow and black bile – so that, for example, eating excess cold and moist foods would encourage the phlegmatic humour, leading to catarrh or excess mucus in the digestive tract. Too many hot, dry foods would similarly encourage the choleric humour (yellow bile), with resulting liver problems or skin disorders.

The mediaeval housewife would automatically temper the character of foods with herbs or other foods: as well as cooking fish with fennel ("hot and dry in the third degree") or beans with pepper, she would have ensured that cold damp fruits were avoided in winter and roast joints of meat were kept to a minimum during summer.

Herb Guide

Amachazuru *(Gynostemma pentaphyllum)*: an anti-ageing, immune stimulant which has been shown to increase cell activity and so act as a preventive for cancer.

Bai He *(Lillium brownii var. colchesteri)*: a nourishing herb for deficient lung *yin* with a sedative action, used in coughs and to soothe the nerves.

Basil *(Ocimum basilicum)*: used in Western herbalism to stimulate and improve digestion, the plant is also anti-depressant and regarded in India as an important spiritual tonic.

Bay *(Laurus nobile)*: bitter and stimulant to normalise digestion, ease colic and wind and improve poor appetite.

Bian Dou/hyacinth bean *(Dolichos lablab)*: used to strengthen the spleen, regulate stomach function and remove excess damp and phlegm, especially in summer.

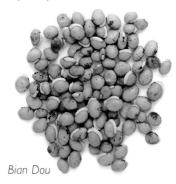

Bian Dou

Black cumin/Eastern love-in-a-mist *(Nigella sativa)*: a popular flavouring for curries and pastries, the seeds are a laxative, digestive stimulant and were traditionally used to stimulate the womb in childbirth.

Black sesame/Hei Zhi Ma *(Sesamum indicum)*: used for deficient liver and kidney *yin*, to nourish blood and lubricate the digestive system.

Bastard cardamom/Sha Ren *(Amomum xanthioides)*: used mainly as an antemetic to transform dampness, warm the spleen and stomach and move *Qi*.

Cardamom *(Elettaria cardamomum)*: an effective digestive stimulant to energise the spleen and kindle digestive energies; also to clear excess damp from the stomach and lungs; stimulates the mind and heart bringing clarity and joy.

Chen Pi/tangerine peel *(Citrus reticulata)*: a rich source of vitamin C used to combat indigestion and nausea and to tonify spleen *Qi*.

Chilli *(Capsicum frutescens)*: a stimulant herb for the nervous system, circulation, digestion and *yang* energies increasing blood flow; relieves indigestion and is strongly antibacterial.

Chives *(Allium schoenoprasum)*: antimicrobial, hypotensive and stimulating but significantly less so than other *Allium* spp.

Cong Bai/spring onion *(Allium fistulosum)*: used to encourage sweating in chills and to disperse cold by invigorating *yang Qi*; eases abdominal fullness.

Coriander/Yan Shi *(Coriandrum sativum)*: stimulating and cleansing herb to remove toxins; carminative to ease indigestion.

Da Zao/Chinese black dates *(Ziziphus jujube)*: used to replenish

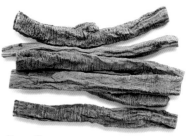

Dang Shen

spleen and stomach *Qi* and nourish blood; mildly sedative.

Dandelion *(Taraxacum officinale)*: diuretic and cleansing herb which stimulates digestion and liver function. A rich source of potassium.

Dang Gui/Chinese angelica *(Angelica polyphorma var. sinensis)*: important tonic herb to nourish blood and stimulate liver; used mainly for gynaecological problems and in the elderly.

Dang Shen *(Codonopsis pilosula)*: tonic for spleen and lung *Qi* and promotes secretion of body fluids; used in similar ways to ginseng but is gentler and less expensive.

Dong Chong Xia Cao/caterpillar fungus *(Cordyceps sinensis)*: potent tonic to restore lung and kidney *Qi* and *Jing*.

Du Zhong *(Eucommia ulmoides)*: sweet and warm, a tonic for liver and kidney *Qi* which also smooths

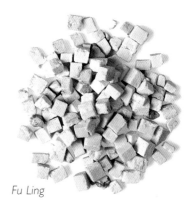

Fu Ling

the flow of *Qi* and blood to strengthen bones and muscles. It is used for kidney weakness and high blood pressure.

Fennel/Hui Shiang (*Foeniculum vulgare*): digestive remedy to ease wind and stomach upsets.

Fu Ling/Indian bread (*Wolfiporia cocos*): used as a diuretic and sedative – said to calm the spirit; also reinforces spleen and stomach.

Garlic (*Allium sativum*): potent antimicrobial; reduces cholesterol levels and the risk of thrombosis.

Ge Gen/kudzu (*Pueraria lobata*):

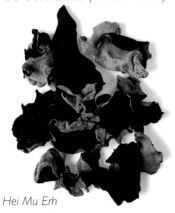

Hei Mu Erh

acts on spleen and stomach and eases thirst and pain in feverish conditions; lowers high blood pressure and will combat alcoholism.

Gou Qi Zi/lycii (*Lycium chinense*): tonic herb, nourishing blood and replenishing liver and kidney *yin*.

Ginger/Jiang (*Zingiber officinale*): warming and anti-emetic for all cold conditions and digestive upsets; dried ginger (*Gan Jiang*) restores *yang* and warms spleen, stomach and lung.

Ginseng/Ren Shen (*Panax ginseng*): potent *Qi* tonic especially for lung, spleen and heart; promotes body fluids and combats fatigue. Traditionally taken by older people in China.

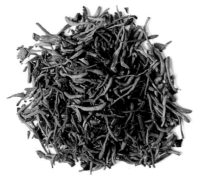

Jin Yin Hua

Hei Mu Erh/wood ear
(*Auricularia auricula*): an effective immune tonic which also helps replenish *Jing* (essence), moves blood, cleanses the womb and eases excessive menstrual bleeding. It is more therapeutic than cloud ear fungus, also known as black fungus, (*Bei Mu Erh*) which is *Auricularia polytricha*.

Hong Hua/saffflower
(*Carthamus tinctorius*): pungent and warm, used in Chinese medicine as a tonic for both liver and heart; to clear blood stagnation associated with painful swellings; and for period pain. The herb can also lower cholesterol levels and may stimulate the immune system.

Hong Zao/Chinese red dates
(*Ziziphus jujube*): used to replenish spleen and stomach *Qi* and are more effective to nourish blood than black dates; mildly sedative.

Horseradish (*Armoracia rusticana*): very warming and stimulating herb to encourage blood circulation and control bacterial infection.

Huang Qi (*Astragalus membranaceous*): *Qi* tonic especially for spleen and stomach; strong immune stimulant which is also antibacterial and helps to regulate water metabolism.

Jin Yin Hua/honeysuckle
(*Lonicera japonica*): cooling anti-bacterial to clear heat and toxins.

Ju Hua/chrysanthemum
(*Dendranthema* × *grandiflorum*): calming herb for liver heat and wind problems; eases eye irritations and clears toxins.

Lemon balm (*Melissa officinalis*): potent anti-depressant, carminative and healing herb to soothe nervous and digestive upsets.

Lemongrass (*Cymbopogon citratus*): cooling, aromatic and anti-microbial herb used for digestive upsets and minor fevers.

Lian Ou/Lian Zi/lotus root and seeds (*Nelumbo nucifera*): the root helps to strengthen the spleen, aids the digestion and replenishes blood. The seeds tonify spleen, stomach and kidney and are sedative.

Ling Zhi/Reishi mushroom
(*Ganoderma lucidem*): regarded by the Taoists as a spiritual tonic to enhance longevity, *Ling Zhi* calms *Shen* (spirit) and tonifies *Qi* and blood. It is sweet and warm, and is traditionally used for general debility, lung problems (including asthma and chronic bronchitis) and for problems related to heart disharmonies such as insomnia, palpitations, forgetfulness and hypertension.

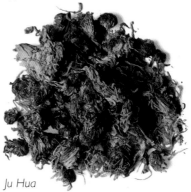

Ju Hua

Long Yan Rou/longan
(*Dimocarpus longan*): raisin-like fruits which nourish the blood and tonify heart and spleen.

Lovage (*Levisticum officnale*): digestive remedy, carminative, diuretic and expectorant: stimulates appetite and eases colic.

Marjoram (*Origanum majorana*): warming, carminative, mildly expectorant and stimulating for the digestion; anti-oxidant.

Mint (*Mentha* spp.): garden mints are of various hybrids and cultivars, all are slightly bitter and cooling for feverish chills, carminative to ease indigestion and stimulating for digestive function.

Mirin: a Japanese seasoning made by extracting the liquid from steamed and fermented sweet rice.

Nettles (*Urtica dioica*): rich in minerals (including iron) and vitamins, nettles are also cleansing and diuretic to clear toxins from the system.

Oregano (*Origanum vulgare*): warming, carminative, mildly expectorant and stimulating for the digestion; anti-oxidant; similar to but more potent than marjoram.

Parsley (*Petroselinum crispum*): a rich source of minerals (including iron) and vitamins which will clear toxins and is also diuretic and antispasmodic.

Rosemary (*Rosmarinus officinalis*): a stimulating, warming remedy for digestive and nervous systems; also carminative and strongly anti-oxidant.

Rou Gui (*Cinnamomum cassia*): a slightly different variety of cinnamon than the common culinary spice, *Rou Gui* warms the spleen and is strongly tonifyng for kidney *yang*.

Sage (*Salvia officinalis*): digestive stimulant which is also strongly oestrogenic and anti-oxidant; eases menopausal problems and has recently been shown to slow the progress of Alzheimer's disease.

Shan Yao/Chinese yam
(*Dioscorea opposita*): especially beneficial for the spleen, tonifies the lungs, reinforces the kidneys and replenishes *Jing* (vital essence); also helps encourage tissue growth.

Shan Zha/Chinese hawthorn
(*Crataegus pinnatifida*): sour and slightly warming, the berries act on spleen, stomach and liver to improve digestion, clear food stagnation and invigorate the blood circulation.

Shi Hu/orchid stems
(*Dendrobium nobile*): sweet and cooling to replenish *Jing* (vital essence) and strengthen kidney *yin*, so helping to combat the effects of ageing; reputedly increases sexual vigour, clears heat and eases dry coughs; restores body fluids (*Jin-Ye*).

Shiitake mushroom/Xiang Gu
(*Lentinus edodes*): effective immune stimulant with proven anti-viral action; contains essential amino acids; anti-tumour and protective for the liver; soothes bronchial inflammations and normalises digestion in *Candida* infections. Traditionally used to tonify *Qi* and blood.

Shoyu: instead of soy sauce, shoyu is used in many recipes. This is naturally fermented and includes soy beans and wheat in equal proportions with a little salt. It has a good flavour and contains no preservatives.

Sichuan peppercorns/Hua Jiao
(*Zanthoxylum piperitum*): traditionally used for digestive problems especially spleen and stomach deficiency with abdominal pain, vomiting and diarrhoea; relieve pain and disperse cold.

Tarragon (*Artemisia dracunculus*): bitter herb which stimulates digestion and eases indigestion.

Thyme (*Thymus vulgaris*): strongly antiseptic, carminative and expectorant; stimulates digestion, eases indigestion and combats infection.

Walnut/Hu Tao Ren (*Juglans regia*): strengthens kidney *yang*, reinforces the lung, soothes and lubricates the bowels; walnuts are used for constipation, weak back and legs, impotence, lower back pain and coughs and asthma associated with "kidney *yang* deficiency".

Wu Wei Zi (*Schisandra chinensis*): sour and warm, used to replenish *Qi* (especially lung *Qi*), tonify kidney and heart; calm the spirit (*Shen*), and strengthen body fluids. *Wu Wei Zi* can be taken for coughs, skin rashes, chronic diarrhoea, insomnia and severe shock.

Xi Yang Shen/American ginseng (*Panax quinquefolius*): tonic for heart, lungs and kidney to replenish *yin* and encourage secretion of body fluids; a less aggressive tonic than ginseng.

Yi Yi Ren/Job's tears (*Coix lachryma jobi*): rich in nutrients (inc. B vitamins) and amino acids; it is a good tonic for the spleen, used to ease symptoms of diarrhoea, clears damp and regulates water metabolism.

Yu Zhu (*Polygonatum odoratum*): sweet and slightly cold, this replenishes lung and stomach *yin* and promotes secretion of body fluids (*Jin-Ye*). It is helpful for dry throats and dry coughs and will ease muscular pains.

While more interest is focused today on ancient Chinese medicine than on the traditions of the West, both philosophies are very similar in their emphasis on balancing the cold/damp (*yin*) and hot/dry (*yang*) nature of our foods. Both also stress the importance of matching foods to the changing seasons and regard diet as fundamental to health.

However, while Hippocrates and his followers argued that one should use food to combat the prevailing characteristics of the season to maintain balance, Chinese herbalists suggest that the foods should actually be more in sympathy with the season, so that the body becomes more in harmony with the prevailing climate.

In spring one should eat more pungent and warm foods to stay in harmony with the upward move-ment of the season; in summer one should eat more pungent and hot foods to stay in harmony with the outward movement of the season; in autumn one should eat more sour and warm foods to stay in harmony with the downward movement of the season; in winter one should eat more bitter and cold foods to stay in harmony with the inward movement of the season.

LI SHI ZHEN: AN OUTLINE OF MATERIA MEDICA, 1578

The problem for those living in conventional Western society, however, is that "nature" and the changing seasons are very divorced from our everyday lives. Air-conditioning and central heating mean that Westerners are rarely subjected to the sorts of extremes which would have been considered normal by Shen Nong, the so-called "Divine Farmer", and his colleagues living in the wind-swept Steppes of central Asia. For Hippocrates, on his balmy Mediterranean island, climate was likely to have been a much less extreme affair.

Apart from this apparent conflict in seasonal emphasis, a "balanced meal" in both Chinese and Galenic terms is one which contains a good assortment of flavours, energies and directions, so that the overall effect on a healthy system is negligible: it helps to maintain the correct inner balance rather than pushing it to one extreme or another.

As well as good quality seasonal food, matched to constitution and needs, a healthy diet should also include regular, moderate meals. Never eat to full capacity and space the meals regularly through the day. The Chinese traditionally eat breakfast at 6am, lunch is at 12 noon and the evening meal at 6pm. In between there are likely to be assorted snacks of rice noodles or *Dim Sum*.

Eating in Season

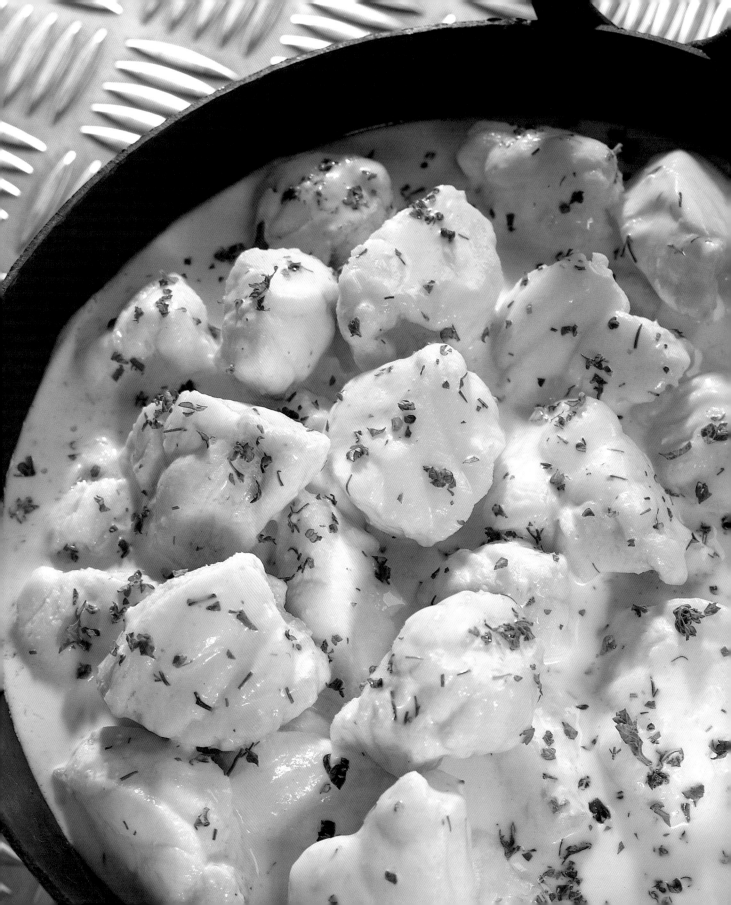

Spring is traditionally associated in China with wind – blowing across the central Asian Steppes: a time of upheaval, change and a need for restoring foods. In Western Europe, spring was a more pleasant time of rising temperatures, lengthening days and rain – although even here "wind" was a characteristic with "March winds and April showers bringing forth May flowers".

Until comparatively recently, fresh fruits and vegetables were always in short supply in the winter, with most households depending on pickles and preserves in the days before deep freezes.

Today, our diets are rather healthier, but spring is still a time for cleansing foods to clear accumulated toxins from winter and restore health and balance ready for summer's heat.

Choose fresh young vegetables, lightly cooked stir-fries rather than roasts or heavy casseroles and eat plenty of early spring herbs.

Meals for Spring

**Monkfish with dill mustard
(recipe on page 28)**

Nettle Soup

Nettle soup is a classic spring cleanser eaten for generations in Europe as a healthy tonic full of vitamins and minerals to help strengthen the body after a long winter.

Winter diets are no longer quite so deprived, but eating nettles in spring is still an excellent way to cleanse the system. Nettles act as a purifier for the blood, clearing toxins, lowering blood pressure and with a diuretic action to help flush the system.

Stinging nettles are a common weed generally found on neglected wasteland, in compost heaps or in hedgerows. When the plants first come up in the spring, they can be difficult to distinguish from other common weeds. If you pull up the plants the roots are a characteristic dark yellow; if still in doubt, confirm by touching the plant with your bare fingers – the stings are very mild in the early spring and are also therapeutic, helping to stimulate the circulation.

Nettle soup should really only be made in the spring, as later in the year the nettles become coarse, unpleasant to eat – and the stings hurt!

Serves 4

225g/8oz young nettle leaves
1 tablespoon olive oil
1 onion, chopped
1 medium potato, chopped into small pieces
1 litre/1¾ pints vegetable stock
Salt and freshly ground black pepper
Crème fraîche, to serve

Remember to wear rubber gloves when preparing your nettles: wash and finely chop them. Set aside.

Heat the oil in a saucepan and sauté the onion and potato for 2-3 minutes, then add the vegetable stock and bring to the boil. Simmer for 10-15 minutes or until the potato is soft and the stock is thickening.

Add the chopped nettles and return to a simmer for a further 10 minutes. Season to taste with salt and pepper.

If you prefer a smoother soup, blend with an electric whisk or in a blender or food processor, then reheat gently for 1-2 minutes before serving. Serve each portion topped with a spoonful of crème fraîche.

Dandelion with Smoked Bacon

Although fresh dandelion leaves are sold as a salad herb in parts of Europe, they are regarded as weeds in many other places, so need to either be grown at home (making sure that the plants do not get to the flowering stage), or gathered from fields and hedgerows. The best time to pick wild dandelions is in early spring before the flowers develop; any later and they are too bitter to eat.

Young dandelion leaves are cold with a bitter-sweet flavour. They are famous for their diuretic effect and provide a rich source of potassium, so this dish would be an ideal choice for fluid retention related to the menstrual cycle. The leaves are also a mild liver stimulant, helping to cleanse the blood.

Serves 4

150g/5oz young dandelion leaves

55g/2oz smoked bacon lardons or streaky bacon cut into 1cm/½in squares

2 tablespoons red wine

2 cloves garlic, crushed

Salt and freshly ground black pepper

55g/2oz feta cheese, cut into small cubes

Wash and drain the dandelion leaves. Arrange them on four individual serving plates.

Dry-fry the bacon lightly in a non-stick frying pan until just cooked, then add the wine and garlic and simmer for 1-2 minutes.

Season with salt and pepper and pour a little of the hot bacon mixture over the dandelion leaves. Sprinkle with the feta cheese.

This dish can be served as a light salad for lunch or with hard-boiled chicken's or quail's eggs and boiled baby new potatoes for a more substantial meal.

Asparagus Quiche

Wild asparagus roots (*Asparagus racimosa, shatavari*) are an important tonic herb in Ayurvedic and Chinese medicine, used to stimulate energy, strengthen the lungs, kidneys and reproductive organs, and increase spiritual awareness and compassion. The roots of the cultivated asparagus, familiar in the West, have similar properties but are more diuretic, while the shoots contain traces of these potent actions.

Eating plenty of fresh asparagus in late spring and early summer, when the plants are available, is a good way to nourish and cleanse the system. Boiled or steamed asparagus served with butter or a hollandaise sauce makes a good starter, or try this quiche for a summer lunch.

Serves 4-6

For the pastry:
225g/8oz plain flour
½ teaspoon salt
150g/5oz cold butter, cut
   into cubes
1 egg, beaten

For the filling
450g/1lb asparagus
3-4 eggs, depending on size,
   separated
115g/4oz thick-set natural
   or Greek yoghurt
Salt and freshly ground
   black pepper

Make the pastry by first sifting the flour and salt into a bowl. Rub the butter into the flour until the mixture resembles fine breadcrumbs. Mix 1-2 tablespoons cold water and the egg in another bowl, then gradually add it to the butter and flour mixture, mixing well to make a smooth, even dough. Cover the dough with a clean cloth and let it rest for at least 30 minutes in a cold place.

Preheat the oven to 180°C/350°F/gas mark 4. Grease a 23cm/9in flan tin. Roll out the pastry on a lightly floured surface and use it to line the flan tin. Prick all over with a fork and bake blind in the oven for 10 minutes.

Meanwhile, make the filling. Rinse the asparagus in cold water and trim the stalks. Cut off the tips and keep to one side. Chop the remaining stalks into 2.5cm/1in pieces and steam for about 5 minutes until they start to soften. Mash the steamed asparagus to form a coarse purée.

Whisk the egg whites in a bowl until stiff. Set aside. Beat the egg yolks with the yoghurt and seasoning, then add the mashed asparagus. Mix well. Gently fold the egg whites into the asparagus mixture.

Spoon half the asparagus mixture into the pastry case, place the reserved tips over the top, then cover with the remaining asparagus mixture. Bake in the oven for 35-40 minutes until lightly set and golden. Serve with a green salad or Forbidden Rice Salad (see page 96) to strengthen the digestion.

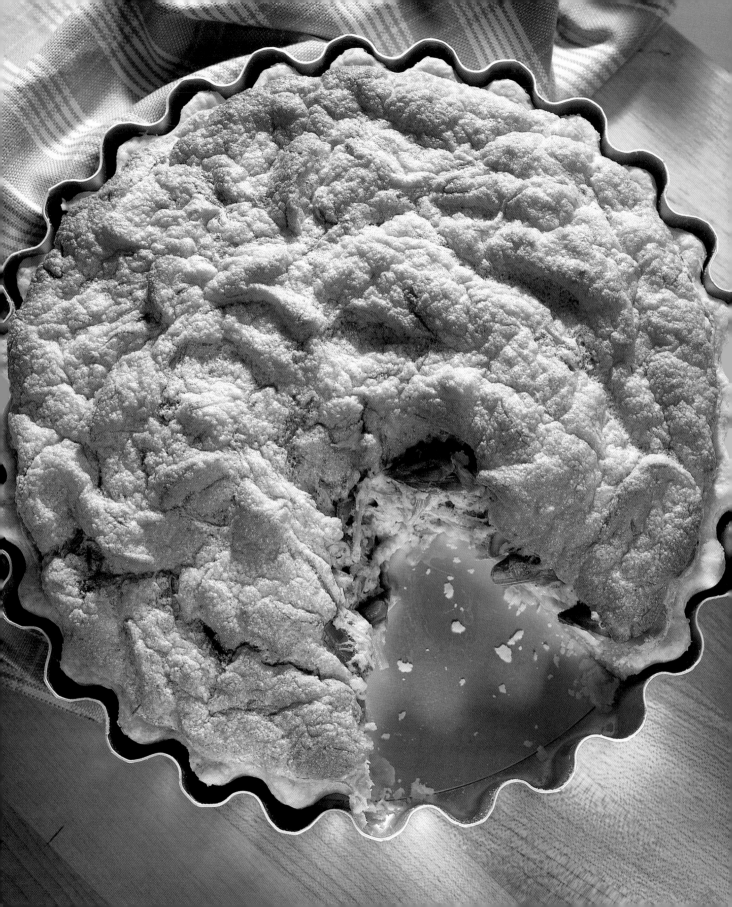

Cold Pasta with Herbal Dressing

In this recipe, the tomatoes – cold, sweet and sour – are balanced by warm, sweet shrimps. The herbs are also warming while the lettuce is cool and bitter-sweet. The overall effect is a fairly neutral dish suitable for changing spring weather.

Shrimps help to tonify *yang, Qi* and blood while the tomatoes focus on *yin, Qi* and blood – together they provide a balanced, energising mixture for spring.

Serves 4

450g/1lb fresh pasta such as tagliatelle or pasta shells
6 medium tomatoes, cut into segments
1 medium lettuce, shredded
225g/8oz shrimps, cooked and peeled
100ml/3½ fl oz olive oil
55ml/2 fl oz balsamic vinegar
1 tablespoon Dijon mustard
1–2 cloves garlic, crushed
Salt and freshly ground black pepper
1 tablespoon chopped fresh parsley
2 teaspoons chopped fresh chives
2 teaspoons chopped fresh basil

Cook the pasta as directed on the packet. Drain, rinse and set aside to cool. When cool, toss the pasta with the tomatoes, lettuce and shrimps.

Make the dressing by shaking the oil, vinegar, mustard, garlic and seasoning together in a jar until well mixed. Stir in the chopped herbs and toss the dressing with the pasta salad mixture.

Serve as a light lunch or to accompany Asparagus Quiche (see page 22).

As an alternative, replace the oil, vinegar and mustard, with 150ml/¼ pint sour cream.

Herby Rice

In Chinese medicine, rice (*Mi*) is classified as sweet and neutral and is especially helpful for spleen and stomach. It makes a nutritious and easily digestible food at all times, but with the addition of warming herbs and spring onions, helps the body to readjust to the changing seasons in spring.

Serves 4

225g/8oz long grain rice
25g/1oz butter or
  1 tablespoon olive oil
1 small onion, chopped
425ml/¾ pint vegetable
  stock
Finely grated zest and juice
  of 1 lemon
6-8 spring onions, chopped
2 tablespoons chopped fresh
  coriander and/or parsley
2 tablespoons chopped fresh
  mint

Wash the rice, drain thoroughly and set aside. Melt the butter or heat the olive oil in a large saucepan and sauté the onion for 5 minutes.

Add the rice, then stir in the stock and lemon zest and juice. Bring to the boil, cover the pan and simmer gently for 10 minutes. Remove the pan from the heat and leave the rice to stand in the hot stock for 15 minutes.

Add the spring onions and herbs and fork these through the rice before serving.

Spring Vegetable Stir-Fry

Eating plenty of fresh, young vegetables in spring is a good way to cleanse the body after the dark days of winter. Asparagus is bitter and warm to re-stimulate the digestion, while the spring onions *(Cong Bai)* are also therapeutic – helping to disperse cold, strengthen *Qi* and warm the stomach.

Early sprigs of mint and the first chives from the garden will add to the flavour – and help provide warming, *yang* herbs as the weather starts to change.

Serves 4

2 tablespoons olive or walnut oil
350g/12oz asparagus, cut into 5cm/2in pieces
350g/12oz mangetout
bunch of spring onions, chopped
1 tablespoon raspberry vinegar
2 tablespoons chopped fresh mint
2 tablespoons finely chopped fresh chives
Fresh mint sprigs, to garnish

Heat a wok, then add the oil and stir-fry the asparagus and mangetout for 2 minutes. Add the spring onions.

Remove the wok from the heat, add the raspberry vinegar, chopped mint and chives and toss to mix. Garnish with the sprigs of mint.

Serve with crusty French bread for lunch or with Herby Rice (see page 25) for a more substantial meal.

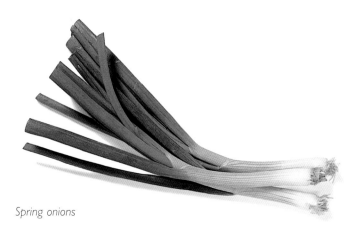

Spring onions

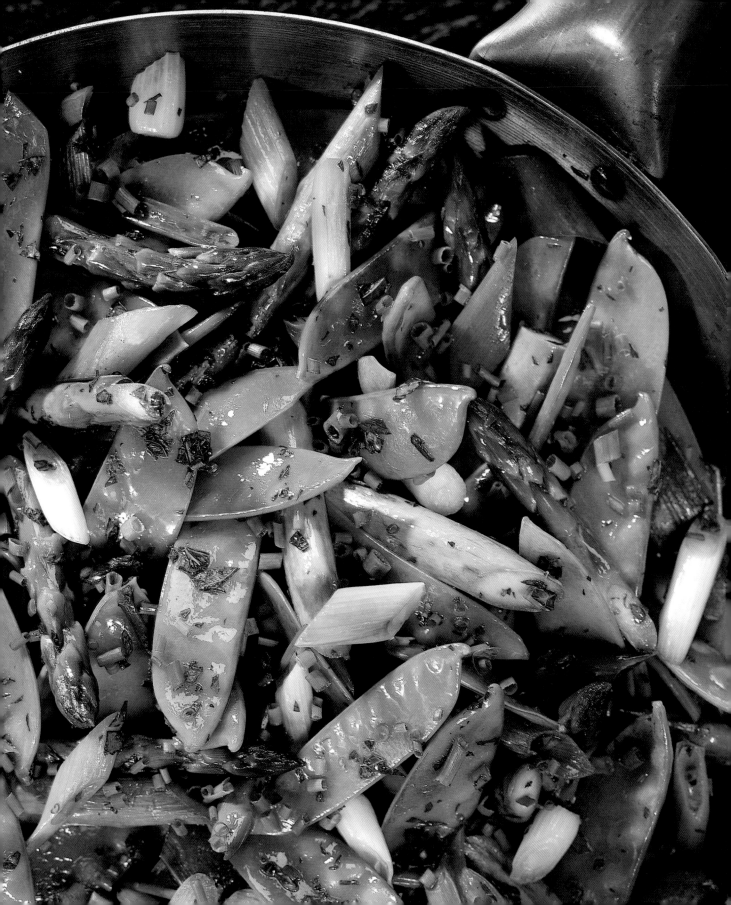

Monkfish with Dill Mustard

Firm white fish, such as monkfish, is ideal to stir-fry as it does not lose its shape and become flaky. It is intrinsically sweet and neutral-to-cool, so is balanced in this dish by some warming dill mustard, which is pungent and heating. Fish helps to tonify *Qi* and blood and is especially good for the spleen, while mustard and dill both help to tonify *yang* and clear cold.

Serves 4

700g/1½lb monkfish, filleted, with the membrane (thin skin) removed

1 tablespoon olive oil (or you can use a dill-flavoured oil, if available)

1 tablespoon dill mustard (see Basics, page 187)

150ml/¼ pint fish stock

150ml/¼ pint crème fraîche

1 tablespoon chopped fresh parsley, to garnish

Cut the monkfish into 2.5cm/1in cubes. Heat the oil in a wok and stir-fry the fish for 4-5 minutes until it starts to turn opaque. Remove the monkfish from the pan and set aside in a warmed serving dish.

Deglaze the pan with the dill mustard and then stir in the fish stock. Mix until well blended and bring to a simmer, then reduce the heat and stir in the crème fraîche.

Return the fish to the sauce and cook for 2-3 minutes or until the sauce has warmed through.

Serve on a bed of plain boiled rice with cooked spinach, garnished with a little chopped parsley .

Summer is hot, dry and can be over-stimulating. In Western theory, it is a time for cooling fluids and fresh fruits. Hippocrates advised "drinks diluted and copious and meats in all cases boiled", as roasting simply adds to the heat. He argued that moving from spring to summer should be treated in the same way as the transition from winter to spring – eat less and drink more.

In contrast, the traditional dietary theory of Li Shi Zhen urges pungent and hot foods in summer – much as hot spicy curries are eaten in India – to reduce the difference between inner and outer temperatures.

Western Europe's more variable summers demand less focus on this need for stoking inner heats – it is more a time for lighter, cooler meals with astringent and sharp early summer soft fruits, to combat excessive heat and balance those inevitable climate variations.

Meals for Summer

Summer Bean Curd Soup

Lemongrass is bitter and cooling to increase perspiration and relieve fevers. It is an ideal summer herb to combat the over-heating effects of high temperatures while the oyster or shiitake mushrooms are both strongly immune stimulating to help fight infections (see page 128).

Bean curd (tofu or *Doufu*) has been eaten as a low-cost substitute for meat in China for at least 1000 years. It is rich in vitamins A and B and essential amino acids as well as being sweet and cooling – an ideal, light summer food. This recipe uses the silken Japanese variety.

Serves 4

**1 lemongrass stem or
  1 teaspoon chopped fresh
  lemon grass**
**225g/8oz packet Japanese-
  style silken tofu**
55g/2oz bean sprouts
**55g/2oz asparagus shoots,
  sliced**
55g/2oz mangetout, sliced
**85g/3oz fresh oyster or
  shiitake mushrooms,
  thinly sliced**
**570ml/1 pint chicken or
  vegetable stock**
**1 tablespoon chopped fresh
  basil or lemon balm, to
  garnish**
Soy sauce, to taste

If using whole lemon grass, slice the stem into several pieces. Strain the tofu and cut into 5cm/2in pieces.

Place all the ingredients except the basil or lemon balm and soy sauce in a saucepan and stir to mix. Bring to the boil, then simmer gently for 3-4 minutes.

To serve, sprinkle with basil or lemon balm and add 5-10 drops of soy sauce to each bowl, as desired.

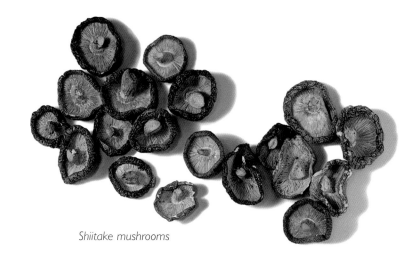

Shiitake mushrooms

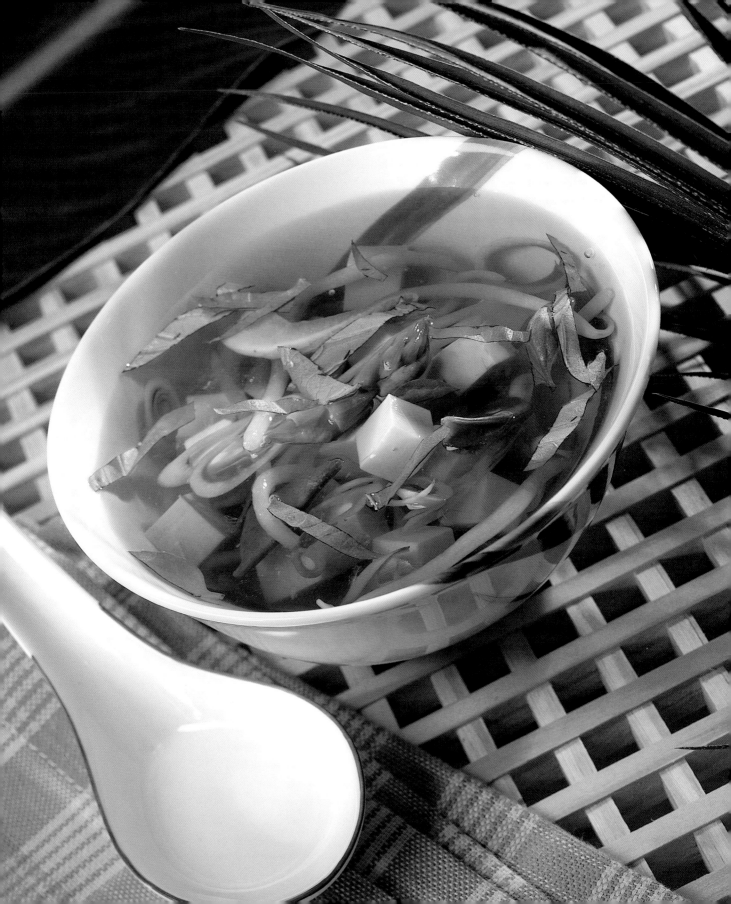

Aduki and Mung Bean Salad

Both aduki and mung beans help to cool the body during summer heat, while lemon and lime are traditional Western remedies to combat summer epidemics – once a common result of poor hygiene. Both are highly antiseptic and anti-bacterial.

Serves 4

For the salad:
150g/5oz aduki beans
150g/5oz mung beans
A head of garlic, cut in half horizontally
1 lemon, cut in half
1 lime, cut in half
2 bay leaves

For the dressing:
2 cloves garlic, peeled
1 tablespoon lemon juice
1 tablespoon lime juice
5 tablespoons extra-virgin olive oil
Handful of fresh basil leaves, coarsely torn into shreds
Handful of fresh flat-leaf parsley
Handful of fresh mint leaves, chopped
Salt and freshly ground black pepper

Start making the salad the day before by soaking the aduki and mung beans in a bowl of cold water overnight. Drain well.

Put the soaked beans in a saucepan with the garlic, lemon and lime halves and the bay leaves. Pour over plenty of water, bring to the boil, cover and simmer for about 1 hour, until the beans are cooked.

Meanwhile, make the dressing, which must be ready to pour onto the hot beans when they are cooked. Using a pestle and mortar, mash the garlic with the lemon and lime juices, then slowly pound in the oil and herbs. Add salt and pepper to taste.

When the beans are cooked, drain them well, discarding the garlic, lemon and lime halves and bay leaves. Toss the hot beans in the dressing and serve when cool, as a light summer lunch.

Prawn and Mushroom Stir-Fry

While prawns, pine nuts and sweet peppers are warming, button mushrooms and lettuce are cool, so together this makes a more neutral combination for summer. Button mushrooms and lettuce also both help to sedate over-exuberant *yang* and clear heat.

To make this dish rather more warming for cooler days, cook 1 crushed clove of garlic or a 1cm/½in piece of peeled and chopped fresh root ginger with the shallots.

Serves 3-4 for lunch or 5-6 as a starter

85g/3oz pine nuts
225g/8oz button mushrooms
4 shallots, chopped
2 tablespoons olive oil
1 small red pepper, deseeded and chopped
225g/8oz prawns, shelled – uncooked if possible
2 teaspoons chopped fresh oregano
1 dessertspoon balsamic vinegar
Salt and freshly ground black pepper
Mixed lettuce, washed and roughly torn, to serve

Dry-fry the pine nuts in a non-stick wok for 2-3 minutes, until they are lightly toasted. Remove from the pan and set aside. Rinse the mushrooms and quarter any large ones. Set aside.

Stir-fry the shallots in the olive oil in the wok until they are softened. Add the red pepper and stir-fry for 2-3 minutes. If using uncooked prawns, add them to the mixture and stir-fry until they start to change colour.

Add the mushrooms and oregano and stir-fry for 3-4 minutes, until the juices start to run. Return the pine nuts to the wok and, if using pre-cooked prawns, add them now. Stir-fry until the prawns are hot.

Pour in the balsamic vinegar and season to taste with salt and pepper.

Serve on individual plates spooned over a bed of mixed lettuce as a lunch or starter, with crispy French bread or a flavoured Italian bread.

Mung Bean Noodles with Tofu

Mung beans are sweet in flavour and cool in nature. They clear heat and toxic materials and are especially useful for treating "summer heat" problems – one of the six "external evils" which traditional Chinese medicine blames for minor or "superficial" diseases.

Tofu or soya bean curd contains four times as much protein as cow's milk. It is sweet and with a cool nature, invigorates *Qi* and replenishes blood. It also combats the toxic effects of sulphur (from pollution) and alcohol, by removing poisons and excreting excess heat in the urine.

Mung bean noodles are available from Chinese grocers and some Western supermarkets.

Serves 4

**2 teaspoons arrowroot
  or kuzu**
**Finely grated zest and juice
  of 1 orange**
**2 tablespoons oyster sauce
  (*Hao You*)**
**1 tablespoon raspberry
  vinegar**
2 tablespoons olive oil
**225g/8oz tofu (one packet),
  cut into cubes**
2 cloves garlic, crushed
**115g/4oz baby sweetcorn
  cobs**
115g/4oz green beans
115g/4oz beansprouts
115g/4oz mangetout
**Salt and freshly ground
  black pepper**
**225g/8oz mung bean
  noodles**
**Fresh flat-leaf parsley
  sprigs, to garnish**

Start by preparing the sauce. Mix the arrowroot or kuzu with 4 tablespoons water in a small bowl, then add the orange zest and juice, oyster sauce and raspberry vinegar. Set aside.

Heat a wok, then pour in the oil. Add the tofu, garlic, baby sweetcorn and green beans and stir-fry for 3 minutes, then add the beansprouts and mangetout and stir-fry for a further 2 minutes.

Pour in the sauce and bring to the boil, stirring all the time, then continue stir-frying until the mixture has thickened. Season to taste with salt and pepper.

Meanwhile, cook the noodles in boiling water, following the instructions on the packet, then drain well. Toss the noodles with the vegetables and serve garnished with sprigs of parsley.

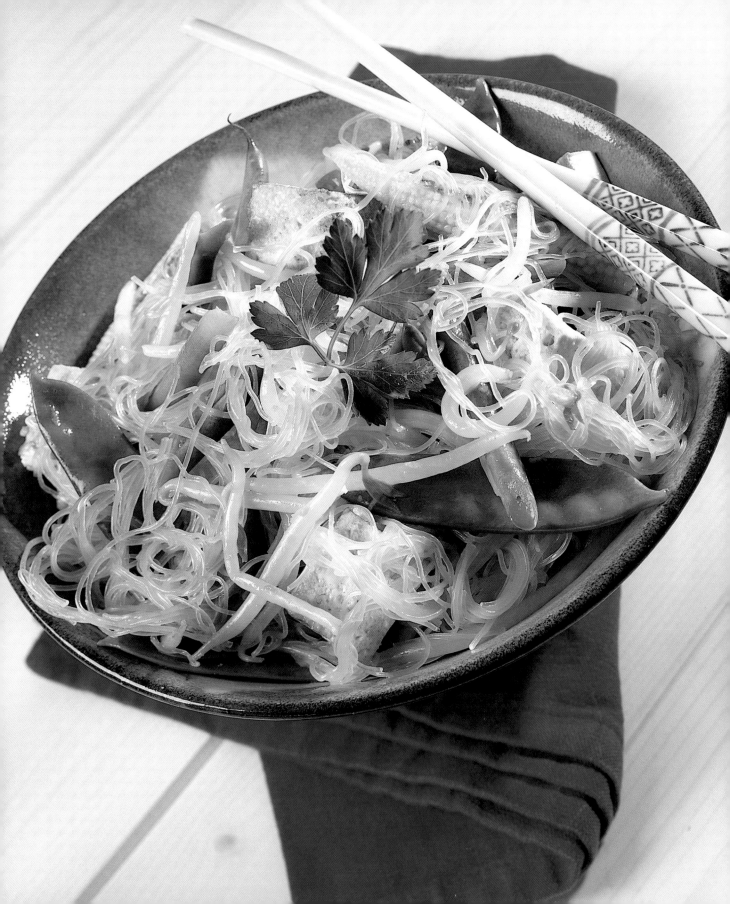

Red Mullet with Tomato

Tomatoes are intrinsically cooling and are warmed in this sauce with coriander, thyme and basil. These pungent herbs are stimulating and energising, strengthening *Qi* and *yang*. The fish is more neutral-to-cool with a salty taste and encourages fluids to help lubricate the system, as well as strengthening spleen and stomach.

Serves 4

2 shallots, finely chopped
1 clove garlic, crushed
2 tablespoons olive oil
350g/12oz passata or
  400g/14oz can crushed
  Italian tomatoes
1 level teaspoon ground
  coriander
1 teaspoon chopped fresh
  thyme
½ teaspoon granulated sugar
Salt and freshly ground black
  pepper
1 tablespoon shredded fresh
  basil
8 red mullet fillets, each
  about 55-70g/2-2½oz, or
  4 whole red mullet, each
  about 175-200g/6-7oz
Seasoned plain flour, for
  coating

Sauté the shallots and garlic in 1 tablespoon oil in a saucepan for 1-2 minutes, until softened. Pour in the passata or crushed tomatoes, coriander, thyme, sugar and seasoning.

Cover the pan and simmer over a low heat for 30 minutes, stirring occasionally, to produce a thick spoonable sauce which should not be at all watery. Add the basil at the end of the cooking time.

If using whole red mullet, fillet them and remove any small bones with tweezers. Leave the skin on.

Preheat the oven to 170°C/325°F/gas mark 3. Coat the fish fillets in seasoned flour and fry them gently in the remaining oil in a frying pan for 1-2 minutes each side. Transfer the fillets to an ovenproof serving dish and spoon the tomato sauce over the fish.

Bake in the oven for 10 minutes or until the fish is just cooked. Allow to cool to room temperature, then serve with a green salad.

Autumn in China is traditionally associated with dryness – a time when temperatures start to fall, rains dry up and *yang* energies diminish as the world turns *yin* once more. For Westerners, autumn can also be a time of "mists and mellow fruitfulness", when damp and fogs start the seasonal cycle of coughs and chills.

Following Hippocrates' advice, it is time to start eating more food, drinking less (to combat seasonal rainfall and misty mornings) and building up inner energies before winter's deprivations hit.

Autumn cooking in China tends to focus on foods to "lubricate the intestines" to combat seasonal dryness, but these can be just as valid in the damper West, as autumn is a time when *yin* energies become ascendant once more and so more moist foods are needed to strengthen and encourage this vital force.

Meals for Autumn

Pumpkin and Water Chestnut Risotto

Pumpkin is sweet in flavour and warm in nature so helps to strengthen the spleen and replenish *Qi*. This is balanced by the water chestnuts which are also sweet, but cold in nature. They are moistening to encourage the production of body fluids and help strengthen lung *yin,* so are ideal for dry coughs and wheezes that are so common as the weather changes in autumn.

Water chestnuts also help to relieve indigestion so, combined with the pumpkin and rice, this is also a good dish for those with digestive problems or weakness. Thyme is a good herb for coughs and lung problems, as well as aiding the digestion of fatty foods and meat. If required, you can substitute (or add) rosemary or sage, which also strengthen and ease the digestion.

Serves 4

1 small pumpkin
3 tablespoons olive oil
1 litre/1¾ pints vegetable stock
55g/2oz unsalted butter
1 leek, thinly sliced
2 cloves garlic, crushed
280g/10oz risotto rice
225g/8oz can water chest nuts, drained and halved or 8 fresh water chestnuts, peeled and sliced
1 tablespoon chopped fresh thyme

Remove the skin and seeds from the pumpkin and cut the flesh into small chunks. Heat 2 tablespoons oil in a frying pan and sauté the pumpkin for about 15 minutes or until it is soft.

Meanwhile, heat the vegetable stock in a separate saucepan so that it is gently simmering.

Melt the butter in a large risotto pan, add the remaining oil and sauté the leek until it is soft. Add the garlic and rice and cook for 2 minutes, stirring, until the rice is sticky and coated with the oil and butter mixture.

Gradually add the hot vegetable stock, a ladleful at a time, while constantly stirring the simmering rice mixture. Keep the stock hot.

After 15 minutes, add the cooked pumpkin chunks to the risotto and continue cooking until the rice is *al dente* and all the stock is absorbed. Add the water chestnuts for the final 6 minutes of cooking, and heat through.

Serve sprinkled with the fresh thyme.

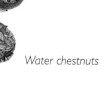

Water chestnuts

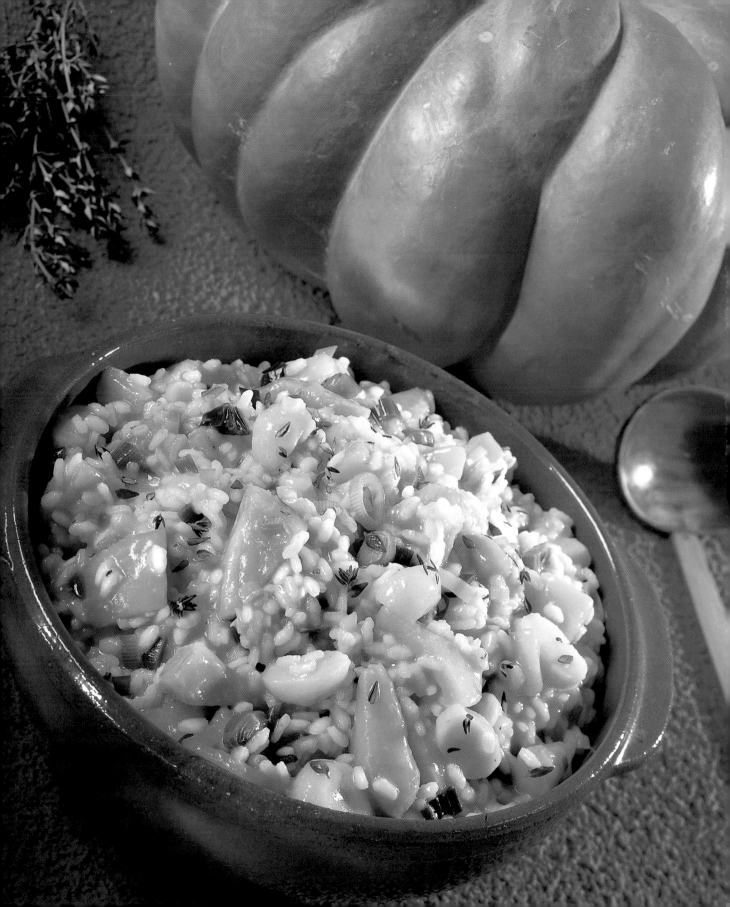

Honeyed Spinach

Spinach is one of our most nutritious vegetables, rich in minerals and vitamins – especially sodium, potassium and calcium – making it a valuable food throughout the year. It is also sweet and cool and neither strongly *yin* or *yang,* so is a good food for times of changing seasons.

In this recipe, it is combined with honey, which is especially beneficial for lungs and stomach, and black sesame seeds (*Hei Zhi Ma*), which are a good calcium source and also strongly rejuvenative to help strengthen the system for winter.

Serves 4

350g/12oz fresh baby spinach
4 cloves garlic, crushed
1 dessertspoon shoyu soy
  sauce
4 teaspoons clear honey
55g/2oz pine nuts
2 tablespoons black sesame
  seeds
2 tablespoons sesame oil
115g/4oz raisins
Salt and freshly ground black
  pepper

Wash the spinach, remove and discard any thick tough stalks and cut the leaves into shreds. Set aside.

Make a sauce by mixing together the garlic, shoyu and honey in a small bowl. Set aside.

Heat a wok and carefully dry-fry the pine nuts and sesame seeds for about 2 minutes. Remove to a plate and set aside.

Heat the oil in the wok and stir-fry the spinach for 1-2 minutes until it softens, then add the sauce and raisins and mix well. Season to taste with salt and freshly ground black pepper. Serve sprinkled with the pine nuts and sesame seeds to accompany autumn stews and stir-fries.

Honeyed Carrots

Carrots (*Hongluobo*) are neutral, sweet and act on the lungs and spleen. They're especially good for strengthening spleen and are an ideal food for digestive weaknesses such as indigestion. The honey adds a little extra lubrication to combat autumn's dryness.

Serves 4

450g/1lb carrots
15g/½oz butter
Pinch of salt
1 tablespoon tarragon
  vinegar
2 tablespoons clear honey
Pinch of ground cinnamon

Peel the carrots and slice them into thin rounds. Combine the carrots, butter and 2 tablespoons water in a saucepan, add a pinch of salt, cover, bring to the boil, then simmer for 10 minutes. Stir in the vinegar and honey and cook for 2-3 minutes, stirring with a wooden spoon.

Sprinkle with cinnamon and serve with autumn stews or stir-fries.

Garlic Roast Potatoes

Garlic is warming and stimulating for spleen, stomach and lungs. Studies have shown that in small quantities it is stimulating to the digestion, especially in the elderly, and it is traditionally used in Chinese medicine to treat "food retention" (associated with sluggish digestion) as well as abdominal pains due to cold. It is also cleansing, detoxifying and anti-microbial – ideal for combating seasonal colds and chills.

Serves 4

2 heads fresh garlic
6 tablespoons olive oil
Salt and freshly ground
**   black pepper**
8 medium roasting potatoes

Preheat the oven to 190°C/375°F/gas mark 5. Cut the top quarter from the garlic and peel only the outer skin so that the cloves remain together. Place in a roasting dish, pour over the oil and season with salt and pepper. Cover the dish with aluminium foil and place in the oven for 5 minutes. Meanwhile, peel and quarter the potatoes. Put them into a saucepan, cover with water, add salt and boil for 4 minutes. Drain and transfer to the roasting dish containing the garlic. Baste well with the oil and return uncovered to the oven. Bake for about 45 minutes or until the potatoes are browned and crispy, basting occasionally. Pop the garlic cloves out of their skins before serving.

Carrots and Parsnips with Sesame Seeds

Root vegetables such as carrots and parsnips are intrinsically sweet – ideal to strengthen spleen and to provide a solid and comforting base as the summer diet adapts to autumn.

Traditionally, black sesame seeds *(Hei Zhi Ma)* are believed to nourish blood and *yin*, and to lubricate the digestive system, so help to combat the dryness which is common in early autumn. They are also a good general tonic for liver and kidneys.

Serves 4

225g/8oz carrots
225g/8oz parsnips
2 tablespoons black sesame
**   seeds**
2 teaspoons olive oil
1 teaspoon minced ginger
2 tablespoons maple syrup
Juice of ½ orange
Juice of 1 lime
Pinch of salt

Peel the carrots and parsnips, cut them into matchsticks, then steam them for 10-15 minutes being careful not to overcook them – they should remain crunchy.

Carefully dry-fry the sesame seeds in a small frying pan for 1-2 minutes, then add the oil, ginger, maple syrup, orange and lime juice and salt. Cook for 1 minute, stirring.

Pour the sauce over the vegetables, toss to mix and serve as a light lunch or supper dish or to accompany autumn stews and stir-fries.

Broccoli and Brussels Sprouts Warmer

These autumn and winter vegetables are rich in minerals and vitamins to help combat chills and infections. They are cooked here with ginger and garlic – warming and anti-bacterial – to make an ideal accompaniment to autumn and winter stews and stir-fries.

Sweet almonds act on the lung and large intestine channels (meridians used in acupuncture) to moisturise lungs and relieve asthma and constipation. Combined with these seasonal vegetables, this dish is also a rich source of vitamins and minerals.

Serves 4

225g/8oz small broccoli florets

175g/6oz small Brussels sprouts

2 teaspoons clear honey

2 tablespoons soy sauce

3 tablespoons lemon or lime juice

115g/4oz blanched flaked almonds

2 tablespoons walnut or olive oil

2.5cm/1in piece fresh root ginger, peeled and cut into thin sticks

3 cloves garlic, crushed

Large handful of fresh coriander leaves, finely chopped

Steam the broccoli florets and Brussels sprouts for about 5 minutes so that they remain fairly crisp. Set aside.

Mix the honey, soy sauce and lemon or lime juice together to make a sauce. Set aside.

Heat a wok and dry-fry the almonds carefully to avoid burning for 1-2 minutes, then remove them from the wok and set aside.

Heat the oil in the wok, add the ginger and garlic and stir-fry for 2 minutes. Add the sauce and simmer for 2 minutes. Add the steamed vegetables to the wok and toss to mix.

Serve garnished with the browned almonds and chopped coriander.

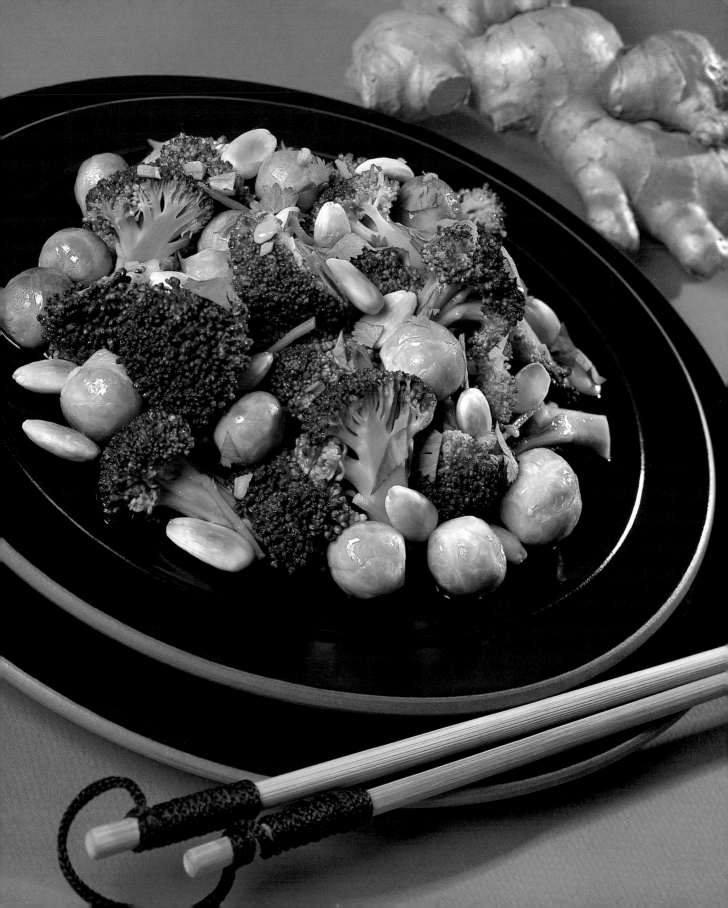

Venison Rolls in Blackcurrant Sauce

In the West, autumn is the traditional time for eating game such as venison, pheasant, partridge and pigeon. They are all warming meats, stimulating and energising to help strengthen the body for the cold days ahead. They can be dry and difficult to digest, so it is always good to serve them with a sweeter, more moistening food (such as honey or fruits) to help the stomach and spleen. Many traditional game dishes reflect this need using seasonal fruits such as plums, apricots or – as here – blackcurrants. The herbs in this recipe also help to stimulate the digestion.

Serves 4

For the marinade:
1 tablespoon garlic oil (see Basics, page 188)
1 tablespoon tarragon vinegar (see Basics, page 189)
½ tablespoon Sichuan pepper oil (see Basics, page 188)
225g/8oz fresh blackcurrants
1 heaped tablespoon roughly chopped fresh tarragon
1 heaped tablespoon chopped fresh marjoram
Salt and freshly ground black pepper
120ml/4fl oz red wine

For the venison rolls:
4 thin but wide venison steaks or slices of haunch
4 teaspoons sweetened fruit mustard
4 thin rashers smoked bacon
2 tablespoons olive oil
275ml/½ pint beef stock
2 tablespoons crème de cassis or cassis syrup
Blackcurrants, to garnish

Mix all the ingredients for the marinade together. Pour over the venison steaks in a shallow dish, cover and leave to marinate in the refrigerator for about 24 hours.

Make the venison rolls. Remove the steaks from the marinade, reserving the sauce, rub each steak with a little mustard and place a rasher of bacon on top. Roll the steaks and their filling to form sausages and secure with kitchen string or cocktail sticks.

Heat the olive oil in a frying pan and cook the venison rolls over a moderate heat for about 15 minutes, turning often until brown on all sides.

Add half the beef stock to deglaze the pan, cover and continue to cook the venison on a low heat for a further 20 minutes, adding more stock if necessary, to keep the rolls immersed in liquid.

To make the sauce, puree the reserved marinade in a blender or food processor until smooth, then sieve into the cooking pan containing the venison rolls.

Add the remaining stock, bring to the boil and simmer, uncovered, until the sauce is reduced by half. Add the crème de cassis, stir and transfer to warmed serving dish.

Garnish with a few blackcurrants and serve with Honeyed Carrots (see page 40) and Garlic Roast Potatoes (see page 41).

Pheasant Breasts with Prunes

Oranges and plums both have a sweet-sour flavour and are cool to neutral. Pheasant, like other game meats, can be warming, so the fruits help to balance any heating or drying tendency from the meat as well as enhancing the flavour.

Oranges can be helpful for lungs, spleen and stomach, prunes for liver and kidneys and mushrooms for the stomach, so this dish provides all round nourishment.

Serves 4

115g/4oz pitted prunes
120ml/4fl oz orange juice
1-2 tablespoons olive oil
4 boned pheasant breasts, each about 175g/6oz
3 shallots, finely chopped
1 clove garlic, chopped
115g/4oz fresh shiitake mushrooms, sliced
1 dessertspoon plain flour
120ml/4fl oz red wine
120ml/4fl oz chicken stock
3 teaspoons chopped fresh oregano or 1 teaspoon dried oregano

Preheat the oven to 190°C/375°F/gas mark 5. Put the prunes into a small basin and add the orange juice. Place in the oven for 15-20 minutes to heat and infuse.

Meanwhile, heat the oil in a frying pan or ovenproof casserole and brown the pheasant breasts all over. Put on a plate and set aside.

Adding more oil if necessary, sauté the shallots and garlic for 2-3 minutes until softened. Add the shiitake mushrooms and cook for 3-4 minutes until these are also softened.

Sprinkle the flour onto the mushrooms and shallot mixture and stir well. Cook for a further 2-3 minutes, then slowly stir in the wine and stock and bring to a simmer, stirring, to make a smooth sauce.

Add the oregano, then spoon in the soaked prunes and add a little of the orange juice to give the sauce a good pouring consistency without it becoming too runny.

Return the pheasant breasts to the casserole dish and allow to boil gently for 2-3 minutes. Cover and place in the oven. Bake for 30-40 minutes or until the pheasant is tender and the juices run clear. If the sauce becomes too thick, stir in a little more of the orange juice.

Serve with Honeyed Spinach (see page 40) and Mashed Potatoes (see page 104).

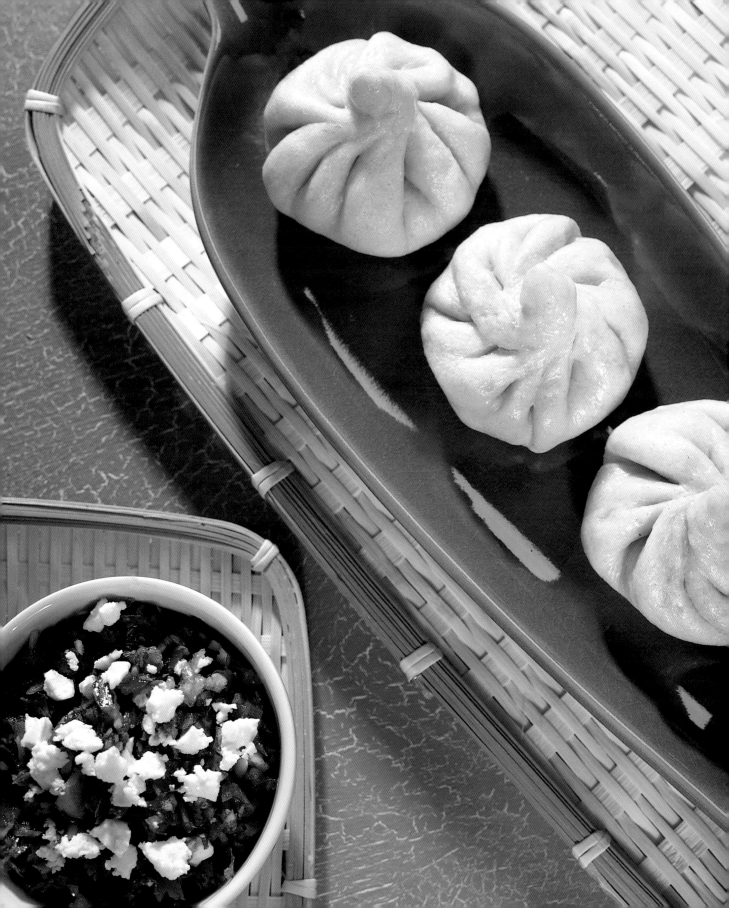

Winter is cold – to the early Taoists who first formulated Chinese dietary theories, it was very cold indeed: central Asia with no central heating, no wonder the early philosophers argued that the best way to cope was to make the body as cold as possible to blend with its surroundings.

Hippocrates thought differently, urging warming, roasted meats and reducing fluid intake to be "neat and scanty" to combat Europe's pervading winter dampness. It is a time for heartening stews, plenty of sweet, root vegetables, dominated by the Earth element, and warming spices. Central heating and motor cars cocoon us from the worst of winter's extremes, so for most Westerners, following Hippocrates' rather than Li Shi Zhen's dietary theories makes more sense.

The period of transition from autumn to winter is when we should eat plenty of energising herbs as well – traditionally this was a good time for a seasonal course of ginseng, to boost *yang* energies for the winter. It is also the time for plenty of immune-stimulating foods (see pages 125-139) to combat those inevitable seasonal chills.

Meals for Winter

Bhutanese *momos* with eze
(recipe on page 56)

Oat Porridge with Cinnamon and *Gou Qi Zi*

Oats are a wonderfully stimulating food for the nervous system, energising and acting as an anti-depressant to clear away winter blues. They are a rich source of B vitamins, and help to lower cholesterol levels and to regulate blood sugar. Oats contain iron and iodine and, combined with *Gou Qi Zi* (lycii berries) help to nourish blood.

    Gou Qi Zi and *Rou Gui* (cinnamon, see page 154) are also warming and stimulating, making this an ideal breakfast for autumn or winter mornings or an evening pudding dish – excellent for the old or weak or during recovery from long illness. Sunflower and sesame seeds together lubricate the large intestine and are good for a sluggish digestion.

Serves 4

Butter, for greasing

225 g/8oz medium oatmeal or porridge oats

570ml/1 pint soya or cow's milk

1 tablespoon maple syrup

25g/1oz *Gou Qi Zi*

½ teaspoon *Rou Gui*

55g/2oz sunflower seeds

25g/1oz black sesame seeds

Pinch of salt

Preheat the oven to 190°C/375°F/gas mark 5. Generously grease a glass or ceramic ovenproof dish with butter.

Put the oatmeal or porridge oats, milk, maple syrup, *Gou Qi Zi, Rou Gui,* sunflower seeds, sesame seeds and salt into the dish. Mix well and bake in the oven for 30 minutes. Check the porridge and stir after 15 minutes, adding a little more hot water or milk if it is sticking or becoming too thick and solid.

Serve with crème fraîche or cream for pudding or warm milk for breakfast.

Chanterelle and Potato Soup

Late autumn and winter are a good time for wild mushrooms such as chanterelles (*Cantharellus cibarius*, see page 130), which are rich in amino acids and a good source of vitamin A – important for healthy eyes and to help prevent inflammatory diseases. In Chinese medicine, the mushrooms are also believed to help tonify the mucous membranes and ease respiratory infections.

Potatoes are an important source of vitamin C – often in short supply in the winter. This soup also contains plenty of *Allium* species – chives, garlic and shallots – which are all warming and stimulating, with anti-bacterial action to help combat seasonal infections.

Serves 4

225g/8oz fresh chanterelles
55g/2oz butter
4 shallots, chopped
2 cloves garlic, crushed
1 tablespoon plain flour
280g/10oz potatoes, peeled and diced
1 bay leaf
4 tablespoons tarragon vinegar (see Basics, page 189)
2 tablespoons chopped fresh chives
1 teaspoon green peppercorns in brine
4 tablespoons crème fraîche, to serve

Wash the chanterelles and trim the base of the stalks. If they are large, slice them but leave any small mushrooms whole. Set aside.

Melt the butter in a large saucepan and fry the shallots and garlic for 2-3 minutes. Add the flour and continue cooking until the mixture is lightly browned. Add 1 litre/1¾ pints water, the chanterelles, potatoes and bay leaf.

Bring to the boil, cover and simmer for about 30 minutes, until the vegetables are tender.

Remove the pan from the heat and stir in the tarragon vinegar, chives and green peppercorns.

Serve immediately in warmed soup bowls, with a spoonful of crème fraîche added to each bowl.

Rice and Millet Winter Salad

A healthy and wintry combination of brown rice, millet, raw vegetables and nuts. Cardamom and coriander *(Yan Shi)* are warming digestive stimulants, while cardamom also stimulates the mind and spirit.

According to the Chinese classic the *Yellow Emperor's Canon of Medicine (Huang Di Nei Jing)*, millet is good for the spleen, pancreas, stomach and kidneys. It is rich in B vitamins, cooling to the stomach, and helps balance the acidity of the stomach, so can help with bad breathe and acid regurgitation.

The warmth of *Rou Gui* (cinnamon), cardamom and coriander also helps to balance the cooling energises of millet.

Serves 4

For the salad:
150g/5oz long-grain rice
115g/4oz millet
1 dessertspoon olive oil
55g/2oz red onion, chopped
1 leek, washed and sliced
20 coriander seeds, crushed
6 cardamom pods
Pinch powdered cinnamon, preferably Rou Gui
700ml/1¼ pints vegetable or chicken stock
115g/4oz sweet peppers
115g/4oz mixed walnuts and hazelnuts, lightly roasted and halved
1 tablespoon chopped fresh coriander
Salt and freshly ground black pepper

For the dressing:
1 teaspoon light soy sauce
3 teaspoons lime juice
2 tablespoons chicken stock

Make the salad. Wash the rice and millet, drain and set aside. Heat the oil in a saucepan and sweat the onion with the leek and spices in the oil for 2 minutes.

Add the rice, millet and stock, bring to the boil, cover and simmer for 30 minutes until all the liquid is absorbed and the grains are soft. Remove and discard the cardamom pods and leave the rice mixture to cool in a bowl.

Meanwhile, preheat the grill to high. Halve, deseed and core the peppers, cut into quarters, place cut side down on a grill rack and grill for a few minutes until the skins are blackened. Remove from the grill and cover with a clean cloth. When cool enough to handle, peel off the skins and dice the flesh.

Combine the rice mixture, peppers, nuts and coriander and adjust the seasoning to taste. Mix the dressing ingredients together and pour over the salad. Stir to combine.

Serve for lunch or as a supper dish.

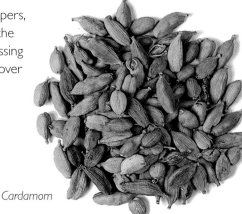

Cardamom

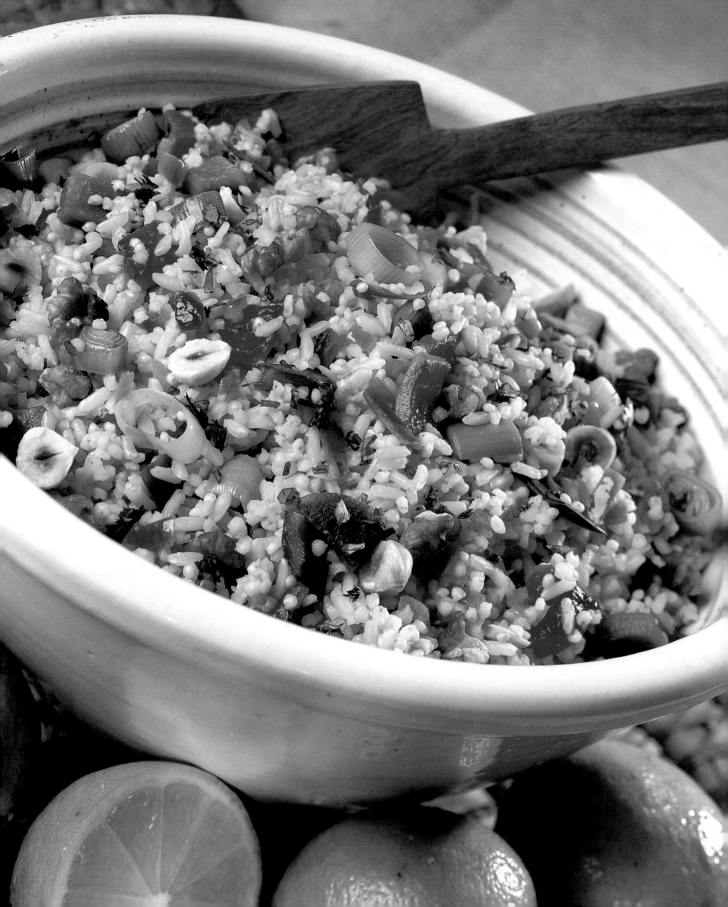

Winter Pepper Salad

Sweet peppers are warm and stimulating for winter, while carrots are also sweet to help *Qi* and *yang*. Walnuts are a good kidney energy tonic so this combination is ideal as a winter warmer.

Serves 4

For the salad:
2 courgettes
2 carrots
3 peppers (1 red, 1 green
 and 1 yellow or orange)
1 tablespoon olive oil
115g/4oz walnuts, finely
 chopped

For the dressing:
3 tablespoons lime juice
2 tablespoons olive oil
1 clove garlic, crushed
Salt and freshly ground
 black pepper

Finely grated zest of 1 lime,
 to garnish

Make the salad. Slice the courgettes and carrots into thin matchsticks. Set aside.

Preheat the grill to high. Halve, deseed and core the peppers, then cut them into quarters. Place the peppers cut side down on a grill pan covered in foil and grill until the skins go black, then remove from the grill, cover with a clean cloth and leave to cool.

Peel the blackened skins away from the peppers and slice the flesh into thin strips. Set aside.

Heat the oil in a wok, add the carrots and stir-fry for 2 minutes, then add the courgettes and stir-fry for a further 2-3 minutes. Add the peppers, mix well, then transfer all the vegetables to a serving bowl.

Mix together all the dressing ingredients, pour over the warm vegetables and toss to mix. Leave to cool, then just before serving sprinkle over the chopped walnuts and lime zest.

Serve with Thick Herby Leek Tart (see page 169) for lunch or supper.

Baked Cod with Pimientos and Tomatoes

Cod, like most white fish, is cool to neutral with a sweet taste and slightly *yang*. It is a good food throughout the year helping to tonify *Qi* and blood, and stimulating the spleen. Adding peppers and a heating herb, such as basil or fennel, helps to warm up the dish for winter.

Tomatoes have a cool nature, so also benefit from a few warming herbs. Modern research has shown that regularly eating tomatoes can reduce the risk of certain types of cancer (including prostate cancer), so it is worth eating a serving four or five times each week – even in winter.

Although mainly grown as a summer annual, basil is often available fresh from supermarkets throughout the year. Summer plants are usually more highly flavoured and – since the leaves freeze well – it is worth preserving some of them for winter use. Wrap 3-4 leaves in a little cling film and freeze; chop when still frozen and use as required.

Serves 4

1 dessertspoon olive oil

3 shallots, chopped

2 large tomatoes, finely chopped

4 pimientos, sliced (or use roasted, skinned and chopped sweet red peppers, as described on page 50)

Salt and freshly ground black pepper

2 teaspoons chopped frozen or fresh basil

4 pieces thick cod fillet or cod steaks, skinned

170ml/6fl oz white wine

Preheat the oven to 190°C/375°F/gas mark 5. Heat the oil in a pan and sauté the shallots for 3-4 minutes until they are soft. Add the tomatoes and pimientos and cook for a further 3-4 minutes. Season with salt and pepper, then stir in the basil.

Place the cod fillets or steaks in a baking dish and spread a little of the tomato mixture over the top of each one so that they are well covered. Pour the wine around the cod and cover the dish tightly with aluminium foil.

Bake in the oven for about 20 minutes, until the fish is just opaque and cooked. Serve with Herby Mashed Potatoes (see page 104) and spoon the wine and cooking juices over the cod as a light sauce.

Warming Lamb with Shiitake and Peppers

Lamb is one of the most heating of meats and, combined with peppers, is the basis of this warming winter dish that is ideal to help combat chills and seasonal colds.

The shiitake mushrooms (see page 128) have a sweet taste, so are very tonifying for *Qi* and blood, helping to invigorate the system to cope with winter's chills. Oregano is also warming, mildly antiseptic, anti-viral and stimulating for the digestive system.

Serves 4

1 tablespoon olive oil
1 onion, chopped
2 cloves garlic, crushed or
   finely chopped
1 small sweet red pepper,
   deseeded and chopped
450g/1lb stewing lamb, cut
   into 2.5cm/1in cubes
225g/8oz fresh shiitake
   mushrooms, washed and
   sliced
1 tablespoon plain flour
Salt and freshly ground
   black pepper
275ml/½pint chicken stock
120ml/4fl oz rice wine or
   sherry
2 teaspoons dark soy sauce
1 teaspoon granulated
   sugar
1 teaspoon dried oregano
   or 3 teaspoons chopped
   fresh oregano
1 tablespoon chopped fresh
   basil

Preheat the oven to 190°C/375°F/gas mark 5. Heat the oil in a flameproof, ovenproof dish and sauté the onion and garlic for 2-3 minutes until soft and golden. Add the red pepper and sauté for a further 2 minutes until they are soft. Add the lamb and cook until browned all over.

Remove the meat from the pan, then add the mushrooms to the pan and sauté for 3-4 minutes until they are soft.

Add the flour and seasoning and stir well so that the mushrooms and onions are well coated. Add the stock, rice wine or sherry and soy sauce and stir well. Bring to the boil, then reduce the heat. Return the meat to the dish and add the sugar and herbs. Cover and cook in the oven for 40 minutes or until the meat is tender. Cuts of young lamb will be ready to eat after this time, although older meat may need a further 20-30 minutes.

Serve with mashed potatoes or boiled rice and steamed savoy cabbage.

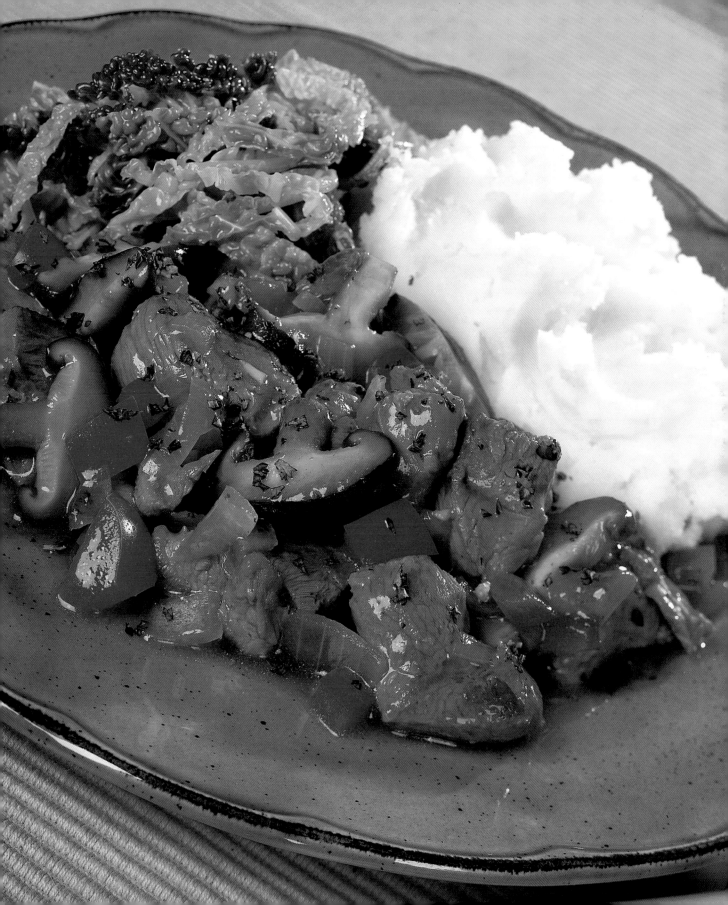

Bhutanese *Momos* with *Eze*

Momos are a type of dumplings always served at Bhutanese social gatherings. The fillings may be based on meat or vegetable, but *momos* are always served with eze, which is a hot chilli relish.

Cabbage is an essential ingredient and one of our most important therapeutic vegetables – anti-inflammatory, anti-bacterial, anti-rheumatic, healing for damaged tissues and a liver decongestant. Lovage also adds to the action – stimulating digestion and appetite. The chilli is equally helpful – stimulating for the digestion, circulation and nervous system and also anti-bacterial.

Fresh chilli (used in this recipe) is less hot than dry chilli powder. Small fresh chillies are often far hotter than large ones – if you prefer a less warming dish, substitute sweet peppers or cut the amount of chilli suggested here by half.

Cabbage is good at any time but combined with warming chillies, *momos* make an ideal and healthy offering for Christmas and New Year guests – helping to strengthen the immune system, combat seasonal infections and cleanse the liver after too much partying.

Makes 24 momos

For the filling:

¼ **of large cabbage, finely chopped**

5-6 onions, finely chopped

4-5 carrots, finely chopped

2 tablespoons chopped fresh lovage or celery leaves

2 tablespoons chopped fresh parsley or coriander

Safflower or groundnut oil, for frying

400g/14oz soft cream cheese

3 cloves garlic, very finely crushed

2 tablespoons soy sauce

½ **teaspoon salt**

For the pastry wrappers:

500g/1lb 2oz plain flour

2 eggs, beaten

2 teaspoons baking powder

1 teaspoon salt

To make the filling, mix together the chopped vegetables, lovage or celery leaves and parsley or coriander and fry in a very little oil in a heated wok for 5-6 minutes. Remove the wok from the heat. Stir in the cheese, garlic, soy sauce and salt and set aside.

Make the pastry wrappers by sifting the flour into a bowl, adding the eggs and mixing lightly. Stir in 150ml/¼ pint water, the baking powder and salt and mix to form a dough. Knead lightly on a floured board until smooth.

Cover with a damp cloth and set aside for 5-10 minutes. This allows the baking powder time to activate, so that the momos swell when steaming.

Roll the dough into a large sausage and cut it into 24 even-sized pieces. Roll each piece into a thin round (each about 10cm/4in in diameter).

Place a tablespoonful of the filling in the centre of each dough round, gather up the edges to a point, pinch together and twist to seal.

Stand the *momos* in an oiled steaming basket. Place over a saucepan of simmering water, cover and steam for 12-14 minutes, or until cooked through.

For the eze:

2-3 large red chillies, deseeded and finely chopped

2-3 large green chillies, deseeded and finely chopped

2 tomatoes, skinned and finely chopped

2 cloves garlic, crushed

½ red onion, finely chopped

15g/½oz fresh coriander, chopped

55g/2oz feta cheese

½ tablespoon extra-virgin olive oil

Meanwhile, make the eze. Mix the chillies, tomatoes, garlic, onion and coriander in a bowl. Crumble the feta cheese on top, add the olive oil and mix well.

Serve the *momos* with spoonfuls of eze for lunch or supper.

Healing Shiitake Starter

Shiitake mushrooms (see page 128) are an important immune stimulant, sweet, neutral and traditionally said to tonify *Qi* and blood, and benefit the stomach. They are ideal at any time of year to combat seasonal colds and help strengthen the liver. They're also good for soothing chest inflammations – common in autumn and winter – and can help lower high cholesterol levels to counter a seasonal surfeit of rich puddings.

Spring onions (*Cong Bai*) are anti-bacterial and used in China to dispel "wind and cold evils" as well as invigorate yang *Qi*. Coriander (see page 120) is an important detoxificant, while the addition of ginger makes this dish just a little more warming to ease winter chills.

Serves 4
400g/14oz fresh shiitake mushrooms
2 tablespoons sesame seed oil
115g/4oz spring onions, sliced
½ teaspoon fresh root ginger, peeled and chopped
Salt and freshly ground black pepper
1 tablespoon orange peel vinegar (see Basics, page 189)
1 tablespoon chopped fresh coriander

Trim the stalks and wash the mushrooms, then pat them dry. Leave them whole. Heat a thick-based pan, add the sesame oil, spring onions and ginger and fry for 1 minute.

Add the mushrooms, cook them for 2-3 minutes on one side, then turn them over and cook for a further 2-3 minutes. Season to taste with salt and pepper.

Transfer the mushrooms to a warmed serving dish and keep warm. Add the vinegar to the cooking juices and use to deglaze the pan.

Pour the sauce over the mushrooms and sprinkle with coriander. Serve as a starter or light lunch.

Sautéed Hen-of-the-Woods

Winter is always a bad time for asthmatics and those suffering from bronchitis and similar chest problems. It is therefore an ideal time to eat plenty of hen-of-the-wood or maitake mushrooms (*Grifola frondosa*), which are a traditional remedy for all sorts of respiratory problems.

Recent studies have shown that these mushrooms are also one of the most effective anti-tumour and anti-viral foods available to us. Researchers have shown the mushrooms to be effective in cases of breast and prostate cancer as well as demonstrating anti-HIV activity.

Maitake mushrooms were once only available collected in the wild, although cultivation is now more widespread, especially in Japan, and they may sometimes be found in specialist delicatessens. Extracts are starting to appear in health food shops as the fungi's potent actions are recognised.

These unusual mushrooms are tender and require brief cooking over a high heat.

Serves 4

4 whole hen-of-the-woods mushrooms

3 tablespoons olive oil

2 cloves garlic, crushed

Salt and freshly ground black pepper

2 teaspoons fresh lime juice

4 tablespoons crème fraîche

Sprig of fresh flat-leaf parsley, chopped

Trim the mushrooms and cut into bite-sized pieces. Heat the oil in a wok and stir-fry the mushrooms for 5 minutes.

Add the garlic, salt and pepper and lime juice. Cook for a few minutes more, then mix in the crème fraîche and parsley and serve.

Winter Duck with Peaches

While most meats are intrinsically warming and ideal for winter, duck is basically neutral, so adding peaches – a particularly warming type of fruit – helps make the dish more suitable for winter. Duck is strengthening for lungs and kidney and these effects can be enhanced by replacing the peach brandy in this recipe with a suitable herbal brandy (see page 182).

Serves 4

3-4 boneless duck breasts (depending on size and appetites)
Salt
1 tablespoon olive oil
1 clove garlic, crushed
2 shallots, finely chopped
115g/4oz fresh shiitake mushrooms, sliced
1 sherry glass (55ml/2fl oz) peach or apricot brandy or peach wine
150ml/¼ pint chicken or vegetable stock
1 heaped teaspoon cornflour or arrowroot, stirred into a paste with a little water
2 ripe medium peaches, peeled, stoned and sliced

Preheat the oven to 200°C/400°F/gas mark 6. Rub the duck breasts all over with salt and place skin side down in a roasting dish in the oven. Cook for 10 minutes. Turn the duck breasts over and cook for a further 20 minutes. Remove from the oven and allow to rest for 5-10 minutes before slicing across into 1cm/½in thick pieces. Place in a warm serving dish.

While the duck is cooking, make the sauce. Heat the oil in a frying pan and sauté the garlic and shallots for 1-2 minutes. Add the mushrooms and sauté for 3-4 minutes until they are soft. Add the brandy or wine and allow to bubble for 2-3 minutes, then add the stock and bring to a simmer. Add the cornflour or arrowroot mixture and cook until thickened, stirring.

Reserve 4 peach slices for garnish, chop the remainder into smaller pieces and stir into the sauce. Pour a little of the sauce over the duck and decorate with the reserved peach slices.

Serve with boiled new potatoes, Roasted Carrots (see below) or Broccoli and Brussels Sprout Warmer (see page 42).

For Roasted Carrots: allow 1 large carrot per person. Peel and slice the carrots in half lengthwise. Place in a roasting dish and add 1-2 tablespoons olive oil. Stir to coat the carrots thoroughly. Season with salt and freshly ground black pepper and bake on the top shelf of an oven preheated to 220°C/425°F/gas mark 7 for 30-40 minutes.

Old-Fashioned Strudel

Apple strudel is a favourite dish in autumn or winter in many parts of Europe. The combination of dried fruits, nuts and apples may seem simply a traditional and pleasant-tasting mix, but it is also ideal for the season. Cooked apple is a soothing and lubricating remedy for the digestive system while the walnuts and dried fruits help to tonify *Qi* and blood, and the cinnamon is warming — ideal strengthening food for cold winter days.

Serves 10

500g/1lb 2oz cooking apples

Finely grated zest of 1 lemon

¼ teaspoon powdered cinnamon (Western-style is best for this recipe)

400g/14oz ricotta cheese

2 eggs, beaten

100g/3½oz raisins, washed

200g/7oz granulated sugar

100g/3½oz walnuts, very finely chopped

20g/¾oz vanilla sugar

100g/3½oz poppy seeds

500g/1lb 2oz filo pastry sheets

Walnut or sunflower oil, to brush the pastry

200ml/7fl oz sour cream

Preheat the oven to 190°C/375°F/gas mark 5. Peel, core and thinly slice the apples. Place in a pan with 2-3 tablespoons water, the lemon zest and cinnamon and cook for 5-8 minutes until the apples start to soften slightly. Remove the pan from the heat and set aside.

Make the filling by mixing the cheese, eggs, raisins and 175g/6oz sugar together and set aside. Mix the walnuts with the remaining sugar and set aside. Mix the vanilla sugar and poppy seeds together and set aside.

To make the strudel, place 1-2 sheets of filo pastry on a well-oiled earthenware baking dish — this should be slightly larger than the filo sheets (normally about 40x30cm/16x12in, but it depends on the brand you buy); otherwise cut the sheets to fit. Brush the pastry all over with a little walnut or sunflower oil.

Next spread a thin layer of the walnuts and sugar mixture over the pastry, followed by a little sour cream, then alternate further layers of well-oiled filo pastry with layers of spiced apples, the cheese mixture and poppy seeds with sour cream. Repeat the sequence with more alternate layers of walnuts and sugar, sour cream, spiced apples, cheese mixture, poppy seeds with sour cream over, then back to apples, cheese again and finishing with walnuts and a final layer of pastry.

Pour the remaining sour cream over the top and bake in the oven for 50-60 minutes until golden. Serve hot with cream or custard, or cold in slices.

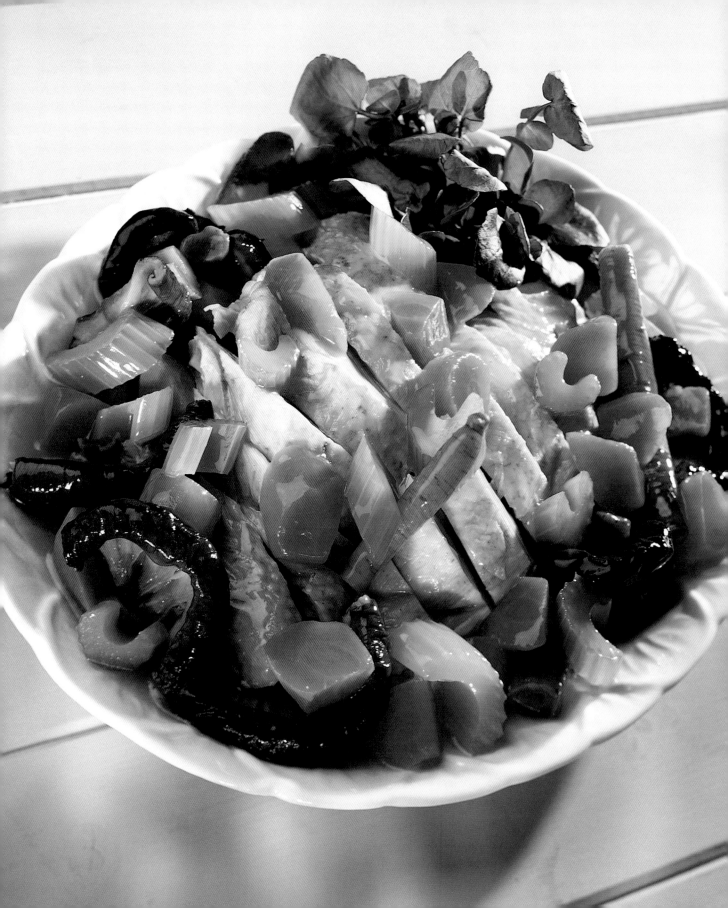

As well as balancing the qualities of the foods themselves, the meals we eat can also play a far greater role in maintaining health than simply providing us with essential nutrients. Many Western culinary herbs, such as thyme, sage, rosemary, garlic and parsley are also important medicinal plants. All of them help to stimulate normal function of the digestive system and reduce the risk of wind or flatulence. They also have a variety of other important therapeutic properties which modern research is now confirming. Garlic, for example, will lower blood cholesterol levels after a fatty meal so helping to combat atherosclerosis and heart disease, while sage and rosemary are both important anti-oxidants which help to destroy "free radicals" – highly reactive molecules formed in the body during breakdown of certain chemicals which can damage cells and lead to abnormalities. Eating these herbs with our meals thus provides much more than just a pleasant flavour.

The Chinese, too, have a long tradition of using important medicinal plants in cooking to improve health. In ancient China, a duck stuffed with five caterpillar fungi (*Dong Chong Xia Cao, Cordyceps sinensis*) and then roasted was a highly regarded delicacy, reserved exclusively for use by the Emperor and his household. Once cooked, the fungus was removed and the duck eaten twice a day for a week or more as an important seasonal energy tonic.

More commonplace, even today, is the tradition of cooking Chinese angelica root (*Dang Gui, Angelica polyphorma* var. *sinensis*) in lamb or chicken stews to eat as a nourishing tonic food after childbirth.

Apart from the potent medicinal herbs that we can add to our food, we must also remember the therapeutic properties of the food itself: many of our familiar fruits and vegetables have an impressive array of properties. Shiitake mushrooms are an effective immune stimulant, cabbage is an anti-inflammatory and anti-bacterial, while our familiar cups of tea are also helping to reduce cholesterol levels and prevent cell damage by their anti-oxidant effect.

The dividing line between "food" and "medicine" is far thinner than many people realise, and taking health-giving remedies in the form of delicious soups, stews and puddings is a great improvement on pills and potions.

Full details of the therapeutic properties of the herbs mentioned in the recipes appear in the Herb Guide on pages 14–16.

Eating for Health

**Chicken *Qi* tonic casserole
(recipe on page 69)**

The strength and vitality of the many sorts of *Qi* (see page 11) in the body are closely associated with the food we eat. Poor or inadequate food weakens *Qi*, while a good diet, with the right balance of tastes and nutrients, helps to strengthen body functions.

Pectoral *Qi* (*Zong Qi*), for example, is stored in the chest and derives from a mixture of "grain *Qi*" (*Gu Qi*) which is produced from our food by the spleen and "nature *Qi*" (*Kong Qi*) which derives from the air we breath. Among the various functions of pectoral *Qi* is to fuel the circulation of blood and regulate heartbeat.

Traditional Chinese medicine has a wealth of potent herbs which have been identified over the centuries as helping to strengthen the various sorts of *Qi* believed to circulate in the body. Some herbs are specific to particular organs and may be helpful, for example, for spleen and stomach energies where digestion is weak. Others have a more general function, helping to boost energy levels and combat lethargy and fatigue and stimulate the mind; a few – such as herbs like basil and rose – have a profound effect on the spiritual aspects of our being.

Among the best known of these herbs is ginseng (known as *Ren Shen* in China). This has been used in the West since the 17th century when the King of Thailand sent some as a gift to Louis XIV of France. It is now, as then, very expensive and it may seem extravagant to use it in cooking but a little goes a long way and it can add a delicious spicy flavour to food – as well as providing a major boost to energy levels. *Dang Shen* has a very similar action and is often significantly less expensive so makes a useful alternative in several of the following recipes.

Energising Body, Mind and Spirit

Power Salad

Quail's eggs (*Chunniaodan*) are known in the East as "animal ginseng". They are neutral in character and have a sweet flavour, so are very nutritious. They invigorate *Qi* and replenish blood, strengthening the muscles and bones. They are an excellent energy-giving food for the elderly and are especially helpful for those suffering from arthritis, lumbago or weakness in the lower limbs.

In this recipe, the eggs are combined with chicory leaves, which have a slightly bitter taste and act as a gentle stimulant for the liver.

Serves 4

For the dressing:
115g/4oz feta cheese
2 tablespoons extra-virgin olive oil
1 large clove garlic, crushed
1 tablespoon lemon juice
1 teaspoon green peppercorns in brine
2 tablespoons chopped fresh coriander

For the salad:
12 quail's eggs
Salt and freshly ground black pepper
2 medium heads of chicory, separated into leaves
Assorted lettuce leaves
1 medium avocado, peeled, stoned and sliced

To make the dressing, cut the feta cheese into small cubes and put into a small basin or screw-top glass jar. Add the olive oil, garlic, lemon juice, green peppercorns with their brine and coriander. Whisk together, or seal the jar and shake until well mixed. Leave the dressing to one side for 3-4 hours so that the flavours combine well.

Meanwhile, make the salad. Put the quail's eggs into a saucepan, cover with water, add a pinch of salt and bring to the boil. Boil for 3 minutes, drain, then plunge into a bowl of cold water to prevent the yolks from discolouring. Drain, then peel off the shells.

Arrange the chicory leaves, lettuce and avocado slices on a large platter, with the eggs in a nest in the centre. Season with salt and pepper to taste and spoon the feta dressing over the eggs. Serve as a starter or light meal.

Quail's Eggs on Toast

Eating energising quail's eggs is an ideal way to start the day as in this "brunch" recipe. They are combined with warming peppers, chilli, garlic and chives, so this would be especially suitable as a hearty breakfast on cold winter mornings.

Serves 6

1 small onion, finely chopped
1 clove garlic, crushed
½ fresh red chilli, deseeded and finely chopped
2 tablespoons olive oil
1 large yellow pepper, skinned, deseeded and finely chopped
2 large tomatoes, skinned and finely chopped
Salt and freshly ground black pepper
6 slices of bread
6 rashers streaky bacon
6 quail's eggs
25g/1oz butter
1 tablespoon chopped fresh chives

Fry the onion, garlic and chilli in the olive oil for 2-3 minutes, until the onions are softened. Add the yellow pepper and continue stir-frying for 2-3 minutes, then add the tomatoes and cook until the mixture thickens. Season to taste with salt and pepper.

Meanwhile, toast the bread and grill the bacon. Fry the eggs in the butter, taking care to keep the yolks soft.

To serve, arrange the slices of toast on a hot serving dish. Place a slice of grilled bacon on each and spoon over the tomato sauce. Top each slice with a fried quail egg and sprinkle with the chives.

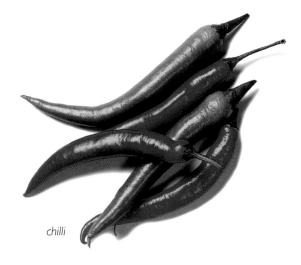

chilli

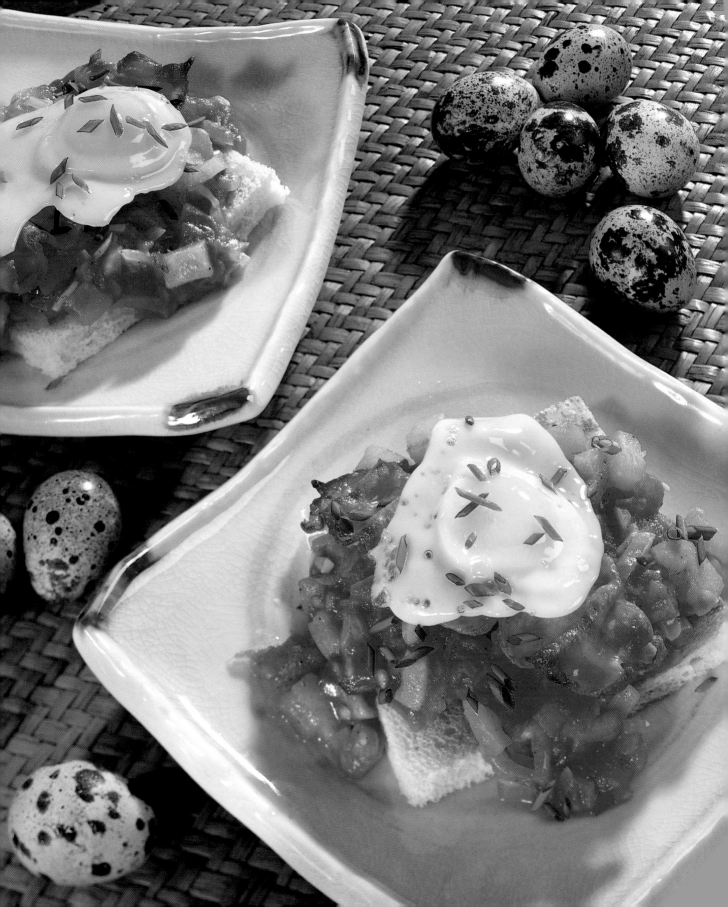

Six Treasures Chicken Soup

This combination of herbs and chicken nourishes the blood, improves blood circulation, strengthens *Qi* and kidney *yang,* and nourishes kidney *yin.* This soup is also good for exhaustion, low libido and to strengthen immunity.

The method of steaming the chicken in a covered clay pot with other tonic herbs for 6-10 hours is very popular in China and is believed to enhance the healing properties. In China, the juices remaining in the pot are drunk as a soup while the chicken is discarded. However, the chicken is still good to eat — as in this recipe. Soup in Chinese culture is said to "lubricate the stomach" so that digestion can take place and it is served either before a meal in Southern China or after a meal, with steamed bread in Northern China.

Serves 4-6

2 spring onions, chopped
1cm/½ in piece fresh root ginger, peeled and chopped
2 cloves garlic, crushed
2 tablespoons sherry (or a medicinal wine, see Basics, page 183)
1 tablespoon soy sauce
1 tablespoon sesame seed oil
2 teaspoons granulated sugar
8 chicken thighs
3 dried shiitake mushrooms
10g/⅓oz *Huang Qi*
10g/⅓oz *Shan Yao* (Chinese yam)
10g/⅓oz *Dang Gui* (Chinese angelica)
10g/⅓oz *Yu Zhu*
10g/⅓oz *Du Zhong*
10 pieces *Da Zao* (black dates)
227g/8oz can water chestnuts
1-2 tablespoons chopped fresh coriander leaves and a bunch of spring onions, chopped, to garnish

Preheat the oven to 150°C/300°F/gas mark 2 or use the simmering oven of an Aga.

Mix together the spring onions, ginger, garlic, sherry, soy sauce, sesame oil and sugar, add the chicken pieces and turn to coat all over. Leave to marinate in the refrigerator or a cool place for 2 hours.

Meanwhile, soak the shiitake mushrooms in hot water for 10 minutes, drain and set aside.

Place the chicken pieces with their marinade, the Chinese herbs, dates and shiitake mushrooms in a clay pot and cover with boiling water. Close the pot with its lid and slow cook in the oven or Aga for 6 hours. Drain the water chestnuts and add to the pot for the last 20 minutes of the cooking time.

Strain the soup and divide the stock between 4-6 bowls. Remove and discard the chicken skin and bones, then add the chicken meat, shiitake mushrooms, water chestnuts and black dates to the bowls. Discard the remaining contents of the strainer.

Serve sprinkled with chopped coriander and spring onions.

Chicken *Qi* Tonic Casserole

This recipe uses *Huang Qi, Xi Yang Shen* (American ginseng) and *Dang Shen* to produce an energising main course that is ideal for exhaustion and debility, as a general pick-me-up and energy booster.

All three herbs are excellent *Qi* tonics. *Huang Qi* is a good immune stimulant to strengthen the defence energy (*Wei Qi*) while *Dang Shen* is particularly good for the middle burner (*San Jiao*, see page 105), strengthening stomach and spleen function. *Xi Yang Shen* is also a good *yin* tonic.

Serves 4-6

1 free-range chicken, about 1.6kg/3½lb in weight
2 pieces of *Huang Qi*
1 stick of *Xi Yang Shen*
2 sticks of *Dang Shen* – or you can use a piece of ginseng root (*Ren Shen*) if you are feeling extravagant!
10 shiitake mushrooms, fresh or dried
1cm/½in slice fresh root ginger
2 teaspoons ready-made Dijon or English mustard
Salt and freshly ground black pepper
3 sticks celery, chopped
3 carrots, sliced
1 tablespoon soy sauce
1 teaspoon cornflour or arrowroot (optional)
Bunch of watercress, roughly chopped, to garnish

Put the chicken and all the remaining ingredients except the soy sauce, cornflour or arrowroot and watercress into a large saucepan and cover with water. Bring to the boil, cover and simmer for 1½-2 hours or until the chicken is cooked and tender.

Remove the pan from the heat and lift the chicken out using a slotted spoon. Cut the chicken into portions and transfer to a warmed serving dish. Keep warm.

Add the soy sauce to the cooking liquid and stir well. If you prefer a slightly thicker sauce – the consistency of a light gravy – either boil vigorously until it has reduced and thickened, or blend the cornflour or arrowroot with a little water, stir into the cooking liquid and simmer for 5 minutes, continuing to stir.

Pour a little sauce over the chicken, garnish with the watercress and serve with plain boiled rice and the remaining sauce.

Be sure to eat the pieces of *Dang Shen* and *Xi Yang Shen*, although *Huang Qi* is too fibrous and indigestible, so should be removed before serving.

Fillet Steak with *Xi Yang Shen* Wine Sauce

Xi Yang Shen (American ginseng) is cool with a sweet, slightly bitter flavour. It is not as stimulating or overpowering as *Ren Shen* (Korean ginseng) although it is an equally important *Qi* tonic, nourishing for *yin*, lungs and body fluids (*Jin-Ye*). It is often preferred for older, weaker individuals where strong tonifying herbs could be inappropriate. It is popular in subtropical Asia for its cooling tonic effect to reduce "heat" in the system.

In this recipe, its coolness complements the intrinsic nature of beef, which helps to tonify *Qi*, blood and *yin*.

Serves 6

For the beef and wine sauce:
6 fillet steaks, each about
   115-150g/4-5oz
Salt and black pepper
1 teaspoon ground coriander
2 tablespoons olive oil
120ml/4 fl oz *Xi Yang Shen*
   wine (see page 184)
150ml/¼ pint beef stock
425ml/¾ pint sour cream
4 russet apples

For the marinade:
55ml/2fl oz *Xi Yang Shen*
   wine (see page 184)
1 dessertspoon rosemary
   vinegar
1 dessertspoon rosemary oil
1 dessertspoon garlic oil

Xi Yang Shen

Smear the steaks with about a teaspoon each of salt and pepper, and the coriander. Mix all the marinade ingredients together and pour over the steaks in a dish, cover tightly and leave to marinate in the refrigerator overnight.

Remove the steaks from the marinade, reserving the sauce. Fry them in 1 tablespoon olive oil in a frying pan for 3-4 minutes on each side. Add half the *Xi Yang Shen* wine and all the beef stock and let it simmer for a moment. Remove the meat from the pan and keep it warm.

Turn up the heat and bubble the mixture vigorously to reduce the sauce to half its original volume, then add the remaining *Xi Yang Shen* wine. Boil for 1-2 minutes to evaporate surplus alcohol, otherwise the sauce will curdle when you add the sour cream.

Add the sour cream, then add salt and pepper to taste. Keep the sauce warm until it is time to serve.

Peel and core the apples and cut each into 12 segments. Fry them in the remaining olive oil for about 5-10 minutes. Add 4-6 tablespoons of the meat marinade mixture and warm through, stirring to coat the apples well but making sure they do not overcook and become too soft.

Serve the steaks on individual plates with apple segments, a little of the sauce and boiled new potatoes.

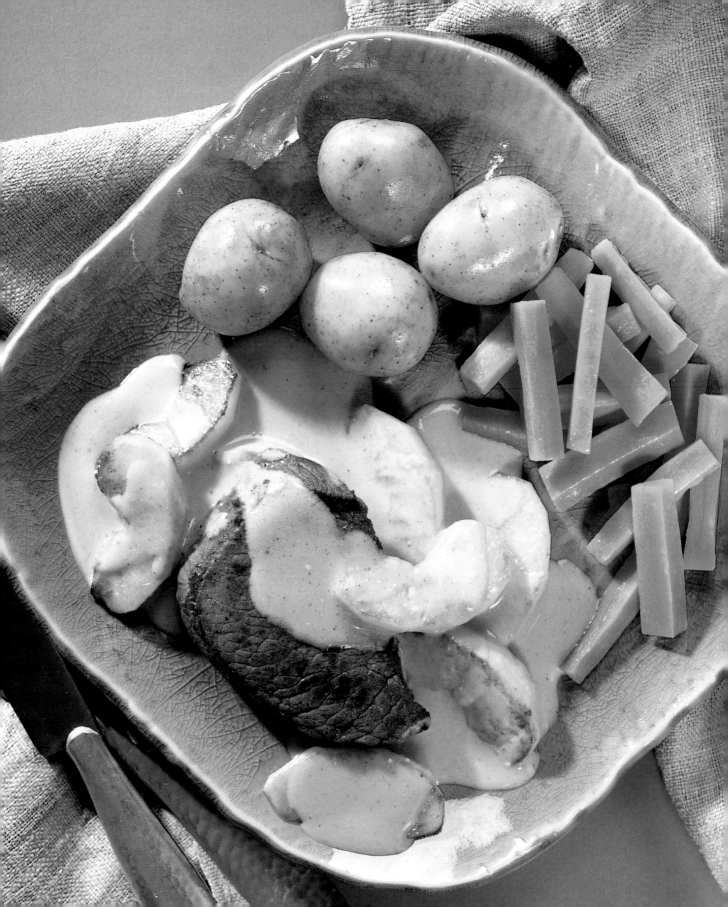

Grilled Sardines with Tomato Salsa

Rosemary is one of the West's most stimulating herbs, rich in a compound called borneol which acts as a energising tonic for the nervous system. Basil is regarded in Ayurvedic medicine as sacred to Vishnu and Krishna and is believed to strengthen faith, compassion and clarity – to clear the aura and strengthen the immune system.

In this recipe, the herbs are used with sardines, which are neutral, sweet-salty fish to tonify *Qi* and blood, acting on the stomach and spleen and strengthening tendons and bones. The cold nature of tomatoes is counterbalanced with the chilli in the salsa. These also tonify *Qi* and blood and clear excess heat.

Serves 4

For the salsa:

8 tomatoes, skinned, deseeded and diced

I red chilli, deseeded and finely chopped

3 spring onions, chopped

I tablespoon red wine vinegar

I teaspoon granulated sugar

2 tablespoons chopped fresh basil

Sea salt and freshly ground black pepper

For the sardines:

8 x 115g/4oz fresh sardines, scaled and gutted

5-8 large sprigs of fresh rosemary

1-2 tablespoons extra-virgin olive oil

4-8 small fresh rosemary sprigs and 1-2 lemons cut into quarters, to garnish

Make the tomato salsa. Mix together all the salsa ingredients, season with salt and pepper to taste, then blend in a blender or food processor for a few seconds to mix well together. Spoon into a bowl, cover and chill for 1-2 hours before serving.

Rinse and dry the sardines. Fill a grill pan with the large rosemary sprigs and lay the sardines on top. Drizzle with the olive oil and season with salt and pepper.

Preheat the grill to its highest setting and grill the sardines for 2-3 minutes on each side or until cooked (they should be opaque but still firm).

Place two sardines on each plate with a spoonful of the salsa. Garnish each portion with 1-2 small sprigs of rosemary and 1-2 lemon quarters. Serve with a green salad and warm bread for lunch or a light supper.

Love-in-a-Mist Crackers

The familiar garden flower, love-in-a-mist (*Nigella damascena*), is a close relative of – although a quite different species and not to be confused with – the culinary herb black cumin (*Nigella sativa*) or Eastern love-in-a-mist. It is native to Western Asia, the Middle East and Southern Europe and the seeds have been a popular flavouring for curries and pastries for centuries. They can often be bought in Asian grocery stores under the Indian name *kalonji*.

Black cumin seeds have a very distinctive pungent flavour. They are a laxative and digestive stimulant as well as traditionally used to stimulate the womb in childbirth. Small quantities of the seeds are also reputed to improve the memory and stimulate the mind. Add to vegetable dishes such as buttered cabbage, steamed carrots or boiled potatoes using whole or crushed seeds.

Makes about 45 crackers, each 3x3cm/1¼x1¼in

1 dessertspoon black cumin seeds
90ml/3fl oz olive oil
Coarse sea salt, for sprinkling
10g/⅓oz fresh yeast
250g/9oz plain white flour
125g/4½oz plain wholemeal flour
1 teaspoon salt

Mix the black cumin seeds with 2 teaspoons of the olive oil and a sprinkling of coarse sea salt. Set aside.

Dissolve the yeast in 150ml/¼ pint lukewarm water. In a mixing bowl, combine the flours, teaspoon of salt, the rest of the olive oil and the dissolved yeast mixture to make a dough.

Knead the dough until smooth, then set aside in a bowl, covered with a cloth, to rise until it has doubled in volume.

Preheat the oven to 200°C/400°F/gas mark 6. On a floured surface, roll out the dough to a rectangle 5mm/¼in thick. Place it on a moistened baking tray and score it into small squares with a knife. Prick each square with a fork. Brush the squares with the mixture of olive oil, sea salt and black cumin seeds and press lightly into the dough.

Bake in the oven for 10 minutes, then separate the crackers from each other and bake for a further 5 minutes, until crisp. Transfer to a wire rack and leave to cool completely before storing in an airtight container.

Serve with Spicy Liver Paté (page 82) or Aubergine Mousse (page 84).

Walnut Roll

Walnuts are warm, sweet and tonifying for *Qi* and blood. They help to strengthen vital energies, tonify the kidneys and *Jing* and warm the lungs. They are an ideal tonic food for all ages, although can be especially beneficial for the elderly, and in many parts of the world are regarded in folk tradition as an aphrodisiac.

This dish makes an ideal energising dessert, served with cream or crème fraîche, or it can be served sliced for tea.

Serves 6-8

For the dough:
15g/½oz fresh yeast
55g/2oz granulated sugar
250g/9oz plain flour
Pinch of salt
40g/1½oz butter
100ml/3½fl oz milk
1 tablespoon rum
Finely grated zest of
** 1 lemon**
1 egg yolk

For the filling:
250g/9oz ground walnuts
55g/2oz chopped walnuts
55ml/2fl oz milk
Finely grated zest of
** 1 lemon**
Pinch of ground cinnamon
1 tablespoon rum
25g/1oz butter
55g/2oz granulated sugar
25g/1oz vanilla sugar

1 egg, beaten, to glaze
Sifted icing sugar, to
** decorate**

To make the dough, crumble the yeast, mix it with a tablespoon each of the sugar and flour and add enough warm water to make a thick paste. Leave in a warm place for a few minutes to rise.

Sift the remaining flour into a bowl and add the salt. Add the yeast mixture and gently work it into the flour.

In a pan, warm the butter gently to melt it. Remove from the heat and add the milk, remaining sugar, rum, lemon zest and egg yolk, mixing well.

Pour into the flour and yeast mixture. Mix together and knead gently until the dough is smooth and no longer sticks to the bowl. Sprinkle with flour, cover with a clean cloth and leave in a warm place for 20-30 minutes to rise.

Make the filling by mixing all the ingredients together to make a thick paste. Turn the risen dough onto a well-floured board and roll it out to make a 1cm/½in-thick rectangle.

Spread the filling over the dough and roll up carefully from a short side, like a Swiss roll. Place the roll, seam side down, on a well-greased baking tray and put it in a warm place for 20-30 minutes to rise again. Preheat the oven to 190°C/375°F/gas mark 5.

Brush the pastry all over with the beaten egg and bake in the oven for 50-60 minutes, until cooked and golden. Remove from the oven and leave the walnut roll on the baking tray until it is cold. Transfer to a serving dish, dust with sifted icing sugar and serve in slices.

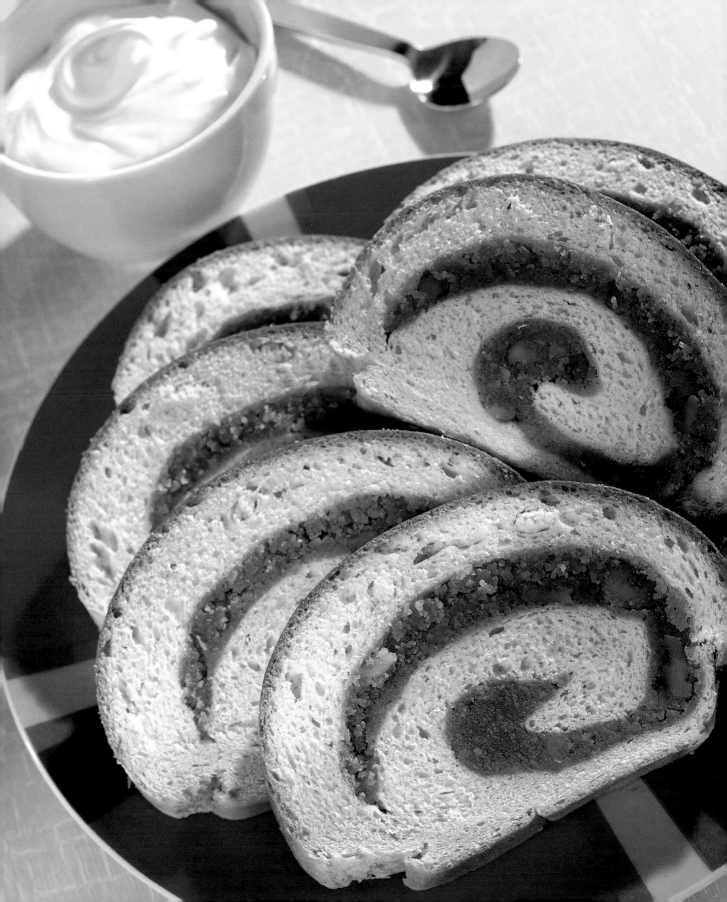

Baklava

This traditional "pick-me-up" from the eastern Mediterranean has become a familiar delicacy across Europe. Its popularity in the Balkans, Greece and Turkey has much to do with the belief that walnuts are good for the mind and also increase virility. In this recipe, cardamom pods are added to enhance the mind-strengthening effect.

Makes about 24 squares

750g/1lb 10oz walnuts (good quality, fresh walnuts are essential for this recipe)
15g/½oz butter, melted
500g/1lb 2oz filo pastry sheets
150ml/¼ pint walnut oil
250g/9oz unrefined granulated sugar
Juice of 1 lemon
1 lemon, thinly sliced
4 cardamom pods

Preheat the oven to 180°C/350°F/gas mark 4. Prepare the walnuts by grinding two-thirds of them in a blender or food processor and finely chopping the remainder. Set aside.

Grease a rectangular roasting tin, a little smaller than the size of the filo sheets, with the melted butter, then lay the first sheet of pastry in the tin. Brush with a little walnut oil, lay a second sheet of pastry on top and brush with walnut oil. Repeat with a third sheet and more walnut oil. Spread a thin layer of ground and chopped walnuts over the pastry.

Repeat this procedure until all the filo sheets and walnuts are used up, ending with a sheet of pastry. The final pastry layer should simply be brushed with walnut oil with no sprinkling of walnuts.

Cut the pastry into 4cm/1½in strips and then cut diagonally across the pastry slab at 4cm/1½in intervals to make individual pieces, making sure that the pastry is cut right through to the bottom. Bake in the oven for 25 minutes, then reduce the oven temperature to 150°C/300°F/gas mark 2 and bake for a further 25 minutes or until the squares are crisp and golden.

As soon as the baklava is in the oven, make the syrup by dissolving the sugar in a pan with 275ml/½ pint water, then add the lemon juice, lemon slices and cardamom pods. Bring to the boil and simmer, uncovered, for about 10-15 minutes to form a light syrup. Remove the pan from the heat and set aside. Remove and discard the cardamom pods.

Pour the syrup together with the lemon slices over the hot, cooked baklava and cover with a clean damp cloth. Leave for a few hours or overnight to cool. Cut into squares to serve. Baklava will keep fresh for 4-5 days if stored in an airtight tin in a cool place.

Rose Petal Jam with Saffron Scotch Pancakes

Rose petal conserves are classic delights in old cook books. Rose petal honey, for example, was made by boiling rose petals in honey for a few minutes and then straining off the liquid. As well as providing a delicately flavoured sweetmeat, this was used for sore throats, mouth ulcers and ticklish coughs.

Roses are traditionally said to be good "for the skin and the soul" and rose has a profound spiritual effect in healing, encouraging love, compassion and awareness.

Saffron is equally potent: regarded in Ayurveda as a rejuvenating and aphrodisiac tonic, it is also believed to strengthen devotion and compassion.

The two herbs combine here as the ultimate teatime treat.

For the rose petal jam:
Makes about 550g/1¼lb
225g/8oz highly scented fresh rose petals
450g/1lb unrefined caster sugar
Juice of ½ lemon
About a handful of fresh rose petals, to finish

For the saffron Scotch pancakes:
Makes about 40 small pancakes
6 strands of saffron
225g/8oz plain flour
1 teaspoon bicarbonate of soda
1 teaspoon cream of tartar
55g/2oz unrefined caster sugar
275ml/½ pint buttermilk
2 eggs
Sunflower oil, for frying

Add 115g/4oz rose petals to 1.1 litres/2 pints boiling water in a bowl and leave to steep overnight. Strain and reduce the liquid to 570ml/1 pint by boiling, uncovered, in a preserving pan. Add the sugar and stir over a low heat until the sugar dissolves.

Add the remaining 115g/4oz rose petals and lemon juice, bring to the boil, then boil to reduce the jam to its setting point. Remove the pan from the heat and stir in the fresh rose petals to finish. Leave to settle for 5 minutes before pouring into warm, sterilised jam jars. Seal and cover as normal for jam.

To make the pancakes, steep the saffron strands in boiling water, allow to infuse for 10 minutes, then strain and reserve the yellow liquid. Set aside.

Sift the flour, bicarbonate of soda and cream of tartar into a bowl, then stir in the sugar. Add the saffron liquid to the buttermilk. Make a well in the centre of the flour mixture and add the eggs and a little buttermilk. Gradually work in the flour, beating gently with a fork, adding more buttermilk to make a smooth batter with the consistency of double cream.

Heat a little oil in a heavy-based frying pan and when it is hot add spoonfuls of the batter to the pan, leaving a space between each one. When browned on the underside and bubbling, turn the pancakes over and brown the other side.

Keep warm in a linen cloth while you cook the remaining pancakes. Serve warm with rose petal jam and clotted cream.

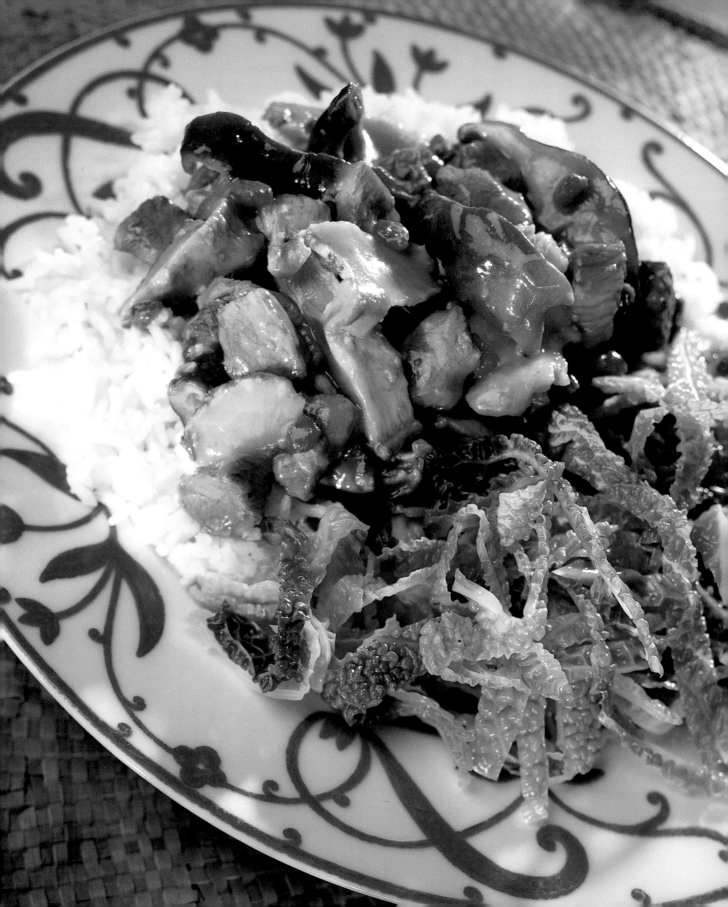

In Chinese medicine, menstrual and menopausal problems are closely associated with liver and kidney energies. The liver is where blood (Xue) is stored so is linked to the menstrual cycle and irregularities here are often defined in terms of weak or stagnant liver energies.

The menopause is seen as a result of the inevitable rundown of kidney Jing and energies during our lifetimes with the various symptoms – such as night sweats, hot flushes and emotional upsets – explained in terms of this energy weakness and the result it has on associated organs in the classic five element model (see page 8).

There are very many herbs used in Chinese medicine to "nourish blood" and these often form the basis of remedies for menstrual problems or for "blood deficiency" characterised by dizziness and cold fingers and toes. The kidney tonics are ideal for menopausal upsets.

The recipes in this section include many of these blood tonics and although they're very suitable for women, many of them are also ideal for men suffering from depleted liver energies as well.

With Women in Mind

Lamb with *Dang Gui* and *Gou Qi Zi*
(recipe on page 89)

Chicken Liver Soup with *Dang Gui* and *Gou Qi Zi*

This combination of livers, *Dang Gui* (Chinese angelica) and *Gou Qi Zi* (lycii berries) nourishes the liver blood and improves eyesight. It is an excellent combination for anyone with iron-deficient anaemia and is also restorative in old age. Both the herbs are nourishing for *Qi* and blood and especially energising for liver and kidneys.

Spinach is cool with a sweet flavour and nourishes the blood; it is also rich in minerals and is another helpful food for anaemia sufferers.

Serves 4-6

10g/½oz Dang Gui
25g/1oz Gou Qi Zi
200g/7oz fresh chicken livers
1 tablespoon shoyu soy sauce
1 teaspoon granulated sugar
1 teaspoon arrowroot
Freshly ground black pepper
1 tablespoon sunflower or olive oil
2.5cm/1in slice fresh ginger, peeled and minced
1 teaspoon salt
500g/1lb 2oz fresh spinach
Chopped fresh coriander or parsley, to garnish

Rinse the *Dang Gui* and *Gou Qi Zi* in running water. Drain and set aside. Combine the chicken livers with the shoyu, sugar, arrowroot and a good sprinkling of black pepper.

In a large saucepan, heat the oil and fry the ginger and salt for 30 seconds. Add 1 litre/1¾ pints water, the *Dang Gui* and *Gou Qi Zi* and bring to the boil, then add the chicken liver mixture and spinach and cover with a lid. Simmer for 30 minutes.

Before serving, remove and discard the piece of *Dang Gui*, but leave the *Gou Qi Zi*, which are good to eat. Serve immediately, garnished with coriander or parsley.

Wood Ear Fungus with Black Beans and Watercress

Wood ear fungus *(Hei Mu Erh, Auricularia auricula)* is classified in Chinese medicine as mild and sweet. It is good for moving blood and cleansing the womb and will also ease excessive menstrual bleeding. It is more therapeutic than cloud ear fungus *(Bei Mu Erh)*, a related *Auricularia* species.

Traditionally wood ear fungus and salted black beans *(Douchi)* are taken for debility after childbirth and are used in dishes to combat pains, muscle spasms, bleeding disorders and slow wound healing. In this recipe, they are combined with watercress, which is a good mineral source for anaemia.

Serves 4

55g/2oz dried wood ear fungus
150g/5oz fresh spinach
3 tablespoons olive oil
1 teaspoon sesame seed oil
1 bunch of watercress
2 teaspoons shoyu soy sauce
2 cloves garlic, finely chopped
225g/8oz can prepared black beans
Juice of 1 lemon
Fresh coriander leaves, to garnish

Soak the wood ear fungus in a little hot water for 25 minutes. Drain and set aside. Wash the spinach and cook in a steamer for 3 minutes, then remove from the pan, drain well and chop coarsely.

Heat 1 tablespoon olive oil and the sesame oil in a wok and stir-fry the spinach, wood ear fungus and watercress for 3-4 minutes. Add the shoyu and stir to mix, then transfer to a serving dish and keep warm.

Heat the remaining olive oil in the wok, add the garlic and beans and stir-fry until they are thoroughly warmed through. Stir in the lemon juice.

Divide the spinach, watercress and mushroom mixture between four plates, top with the black beans and garnish with coriander leaves. Serve as a light lunch or with plain boiled rice for a more substantial supper dish.

Spicy Liver Pâté

Liver is an excellent food to replenish blood, tonify the liver and improve eyesight. It is particularly useful for problems associated with "liver blood deficiency", which in Chinese theory can be linked to menstrual irregularities as well as night blindness and cataracts.

With all types of offal it is important to use good quality meat: this is especially true of liver as it tends to filter and concentrate pollutant chemicals. Use organically reared liver wherever possible. In this recipe, calf, lamb or chicken livers can be used.

Serves 6
55g/2oz butter
85g/3oz plain flour
275ml/½ pint milk
225g/8oz minced pork
450g/1lb minced liver
1 onion, finely chopped
3 cloves garlic, crushed
1 large red or green chilli, deseeded and finely chopped
25g/1oz *Gou Qi Zi* (lycii berries), washed
3 eggs, beaten
1 level teaspoon salt
1 teaspoon freshly ground black pepper
2 tablespoons *Dang Gui* brandy (see page 185)

Preheat the oven to 170°C/325°F/gas mark 3. Melt the butter in a saucepan, add the flour and stir to make a roux. Gradually stir in the milk and bring to the boil, stirring constantly to make a smooth, thick sauce.

Add the minced pork and stir well, then remove the pan from the heat. Add the minced liver, onion, garlic, chilli and *Gou Qi Zi*, then the eggs. Mix well. Season with salt and pepper, then add the brandy and stir to make a smooth paste.

Grease a 900g/2lb loaf tin well. Spoon the liver mixture into the tin and press down firmly. Stand the tin in a roasting dish and half-fill the roasting dish with hot water. Bake the pâté in the oven for 1 hour.

When cooked, remove from the oven and leave to cool in the tin. Once the pâté is cold, turn out onto a plate and either serve immediately or chill before serving.

Serve in slices with French bread and green salad for lunch or with toast as a starter. This pâté is also ideal spread on Love-in-the-Mist Crackers (see page 73) for canapés.

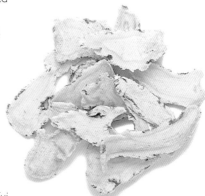

Dang Gui

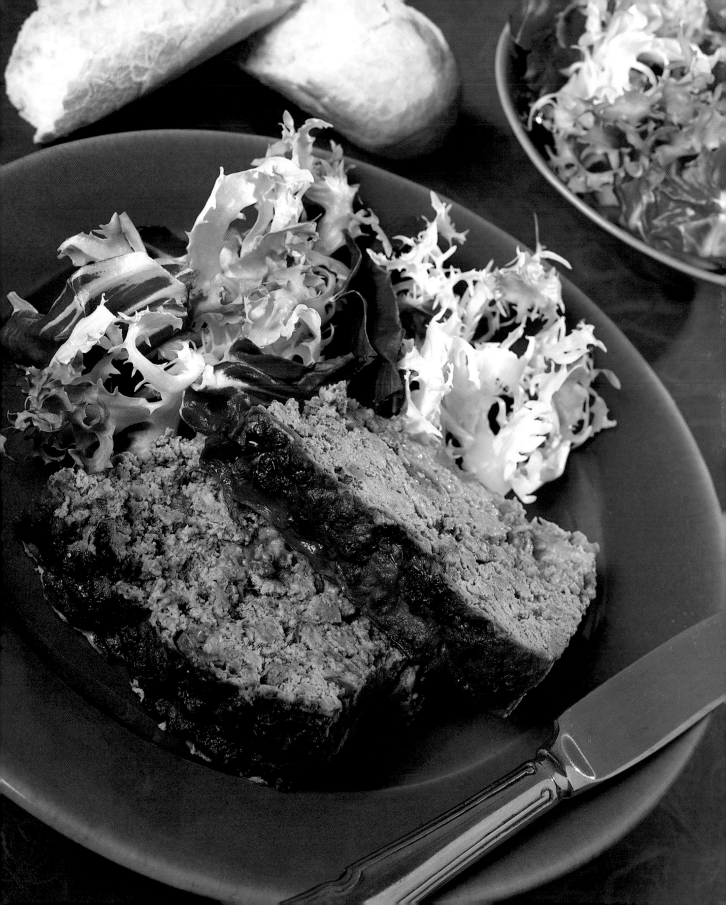

Aubergine Mousse

Aubergine or eggplant is an effective food to ease excess *yang* and to improve blood circulation. It is ideal for clearing "stagnant blood" in the lower burner or lower *Jiao* (see page 105), which is often associated with ovarian cysts and menstrual disorders.

Blood stagnation or stasis is one of the most significant causes of internal illness in Chinese theory. It is seen as some sort of blockage in the normal circulation, but that doesn't always equate with the Western concept of a blood clot or thrombosis. *Qi* stagnation or deficiency is believed to interfere with normal blood flow and blood stasis can also be caused by "cold", causing it to congeal and slow down; by "heat", increasing the flow and leading to haemorrhage; or by injuries and wounds. Blood stasis is often associated with a stabbing pain, enlargement or swelling of the body organs, or some sort of bleeding.

By stimulating the *Qi* and blood, aubergines can help to ease these "stagnant blood" problems. This recipe includes chilli which also helps to stimulate the circulation.

Serves 4-6

3-4 large aubergines (about 1kg/2¼lb total weight)

2 teaspoons chilli oil (see Basics, page 188)

1 tablespoon coriander oil (see Basics, page 188)

1 onion, chopped

3-5 cloves garlic, crushed

150ml/¼ pint sour cream

2 tablespoons chopped fresh coriander, to garnish

Preheat the oven to 180°C/350°F/gas mark 4. Rinse the aubergines and prick them all over with a fork. Place them on a baking sheet and bake in the oven for about 1 hour, until tender. Allow the cooked aubergines to cool slightly, then peel and roughly chop them.

Heat the flavoured oils in a frying pan and sauté the onion and garlic for 3-4 minutes, until soft and golden.

Transfer to a mixing bowl and add the chopped aubergines and sour cream, mixing well. Mash well to form a smooth paste or blend in a blender or food processor until smooth.

Spoon into a bowl and garnish with chopped coriander. Serve with chunks of French bread and a green salad for lunch or with melba toast as a starter.

Stuffed *Lian Ou*

Lian Ou (lotus root) is a sweet and neutral food which helps to nourish blood and clear heat and stagnation. It is ideal for anaemic, blood-deficient women (or indeed men). *Lian Ou* also helps strengthen the lungs, so is useful for lingering coughs and weakness following flu.

Glutinous rice (*Ruomi*) is a highly polished, sweet type of rice which is regarded as a luxury in China. It tonifies *Qi* and blood and helps reinforce the action of the lotus root in strengthening the lungs. Parsley is also rich in minerals and vitamins so will also help in cases of debility and anaemia.

Serves 2

55g/2oz glutinous rice
2 fresh lotus roots
1 tablespoon chopped fresh
   parsley, to garnish
Granulated sugar, to taste
   (optional)

Wash the glutinous rice carefully, then drain. Remove the outer skin of the lotus roots using a vegetable peeler and then use chopsticks to fill up the lotus root holes with the glutinous rice.

Place the stuffed roots in a saucepan and cover with water. Cover the pan, bring to the boil and simmer very gently for 1 hour, making sure that the water continues to cover the roots and rice – add more liquid if necessary.

Test that the rice is cooked deep inside the lotus roots and use a chopstick to check that the lotus flesh has slightly softened. It may need to cook a little longer depending on the size and freshness of the lotus root.

Remove the pan from the heat and transfer the stuffed roots to a serving dish. Slice the lotus roots thickly and sprinkle with parsley. The roots are slightly bitter so sprinkle them with sugar if you like.

Chicken Drumsticks with Black Beans and Red and Black Dates

This casserole is a tonic for the heart and helps the blood circulation. It also makes a good blood tonic for women and will also help strengthen the digestion. Dates are an important tonic for spleen and stomach *Qi* and also help to nourish the blood. Watercress is rich in minerals and vitamins and also helps to restore flagging energies. Black beans tonify the blood and stimulate its circulation; they also help to relieve stifness in joints caused by "wind", one of the external evils the Chinese blame for many types of disease, including rheumatism and arthritis. The combination helps to build blood and energy as well as aiding digestion.

Serves 3
115g/4oz dried black beans
6 chicken drumsticks
10 *Hong Zao* (red dates)
10 *Da Zao* (black dates)
3 slices peeled fresh root ginger, each about 1cm/½in
3 cloves garlic, peeled but left whole
Sea salt and freshly ground black pepper
1 heaped teaspoon arrowroot (optional)
Watercress, roughly chopped
Water or chicken stock

Fry the black beans without oil in a non-stick pan until they jump, then wash them thoroughly in a sieve under running water. Drain well.

Put the beans and all the remaining ingredients except the arrowroot and the watercress into a saucepan and cover with water or stock. Bring to the boil, cover the pan and simmer gently for 3 hours.

By this time the chicken will have fallen from the drumsticks, so remove the bones and skin and transfer the meat, dates and beans to a warmed serving dish using a slotted spoon. Keep warm.

If necessary, boil the liquid remaining in the pan vigorously to reduce and thicken or dissolve the arrowroot in a little water, add to the juices in the pan and simmer for 5 minutes, stirring. Adjust the seasoning to taste.

Pour the sauce over the chicken and date stew, garnish with watercress and serve with plain boiled rice.

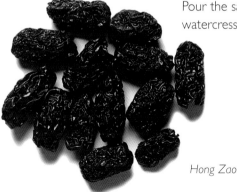

Hong Zao

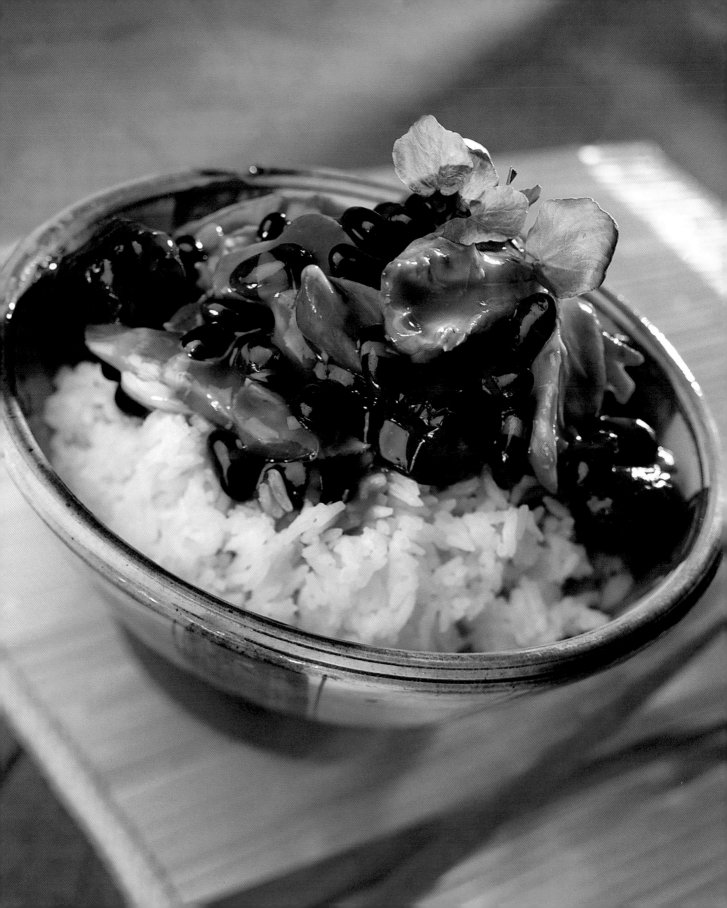

Roast Pork with Salted Black Beans and Ginger

This dish will help to nourish blood and strengthen *yin,* so is ideal for women – especially those suffering from heavy menstrual bleeding in the run-up to the menopause.

Black beans (*Douchi*) are usually sold loose in Chinese supermarkets or, increasingly, vacuum-packed in Western-style cartons. They are sometimes described as a forerunner to soy sauce with the soft fermented beans adding a similar flavour. They will last for up to 5 years if stored in a cool, dark place.

In this recipe, the beans help to detoxify the system and clear heat, while the ginger will stimulate the digestion.

Serves 6-8

5cm/2in piece fresh root ginger, peeled and finely chopped

3 cloves garlic, peeled

2 tablespoons fermented and salted black beans, finely chopped

2 tablespoons sesame oil

2 tablespoons rice wine or sherry

1.3kg/3lb pork joint, either leg or loin – ask your butcher to score it for you

Preheat the oven to 240°C/475°F/gas mark 9. Place the ginger, garlic and black beans in a pestle and mortar and crush to a paste. Add the sesame oil and rice wine or sherry and mix well.

If the skin of the pork joint has not been scored, use the tip of a sharp knife and cut into the skin all over with quick jerky movements. Rub the paste into the joint and into any cavities until the pork is well covered all over.

Place the pork in a roasting tin and roast in the oven for 20 minutes. Reduce the oven temperature to 190°C/375°F/gas mark 5 and continue roasting for a further 1¾ hours, or until the pork is well cooked (allow 35 minutes per 450g/1lb of raw meat).

When cooked, remove the joint from the oven and allow it to "rest" for 15 minutes before carving. Carve the joint and serve the slices of pork on a bed of spinach noodles.

Lamb with *Dang Gui* and *Gou Qi Zi*

This hearty winter dish uses *Dang Gui* (Chinese angelica) and *Gou Qi Zi* (lycii berries) which are important herbs to help nourish the blood and invigorate the circulation.

It is a strengthening tonic dish for women with a tendency for anaemia or menstrual irregularities, and is also ideal for anyone suffering from over-work or exhaustion. It makes a restorative meal for any condition associated with blood stagnation (see page 84) or deficiency – the sort of health problems which may involve poor circulation or heart irregularities.

Serves 4

450g/1lb lean lamb
12 shiitake mushrooms (fresh or dried)
2 tablespoons olive oil
3 slices peeled fresh ginger root, each about 1cm/½in
2 cloves garlic, crushed
10g/⅓oz *Dang Gui*
10g/⅓oz *Gou Qi Zi*
1 litre/1¾ pints water or vegetable stock
Sea salt and freshly ground black pepper

Cut the lamb into 1cm/½in cubes and set aside. If using dried shiitake mushrooms, soak them for 30 minutes in warm water. Drain and reserve the liquid to add to the stew. Slice the soaked or fresh mushrooms.

Heat the oil in a wok or large saucepan and stir-fry the lamb with the ginger for 1 minute or until lightly browned.

Add the garlic, mushrooms, *Dang Gui*, *Gou Qi Zi*, water or stock and seasoning. Cover the wok or saucepan with a lid, bring to the boil and simmer gently for 2½ hours until the lamb is cooked and tender.

Serve the stew with plenty of plain boiled rice or crusty bread and cooked carrots or steamed savoy cabbage.

Remove the *Dang Gui* before serving, but eat the pieces of *Gou Qi Zi*.

Carrot Cake with *Gou Qi Zi* and *Long Yan Rou*

This recipe nourishes blood and between them, the *Gou Qi Zi* (lycii berries) and *Long Yan Rou* (longan) help to nourish liver, spleen and kidneys. The *Long Yan Rou* is especially calming to the spirit, while the *Gou Qi Zi* is said to "brighten the spirit and promote cheerfulness".

The walnuts tonify and warm the kidneys while also lubricating a sluggish digestion. The carrots are sweet and neutral to strengthen the spleen and help digestion by removing stagnation of food. Carrots strengthen both the kidney *yin* and *yang* if eaten over a long period of time. They help digestion of the sweeter *Gou Qi Zi* and *Long Yan Rou*.

This cake makes an excellent blood tonic for women and the emphasis on kidney energy also makes it extremely helpful for older people.

Serves 8-10

For the cake:
225g/8oz unsalted butter
175g/6oz soft brown sugar
4 eggs
Finely grated zest of 1 orange
4 teaspoons lemon juice
85g/3oz wholemeal self-raising flour
85g/3oz white self-raising flour
1 teaspoon baking powder
55g/2oz *Gou Qi Zi*, washed
55g/2oz *Long Yan Rou*, washed
55g/2oz ground almonds
150g/5oz walnut pieces, chopped (reserve a few for decoration)
350g/12oz organic carrots, peeled and grated

For the icing:
225g/8oz cream cheese
2 teaspoons maple syrup
1 teaspoon lemon juice

Preheat the oven to 180°C/350°F/gas mark 4. Grease and line a deep 20cm/8in round cake tin.

Allow the butter to soften at room temperature and cream it with the sugar in a bowl until pale and fluffy.

Beat the eggs well and then gradually beat them into the creamed mixture. Add the orange zest and lemon juice and mix well.

Sift the flours and baking powder together and fold into the creamed mixture. Stir in the *Gou Qi Zi, Long Yan Rou,* almonds, walnuts and carrots, mixing well. Pour into the prepared tin and level the surface.

Bake in the oven for 1½ hours until cooked and golden. Cover the top with foil after 1 hour if it starts to brown. Turn out onto a wire rack to cool.

Make the icing by mixing the cream cheese, maple syrup and lemon juice together and spread over the top of the cold cake. Sprinkle with the reserved walnuts.

Gou Qi Zi

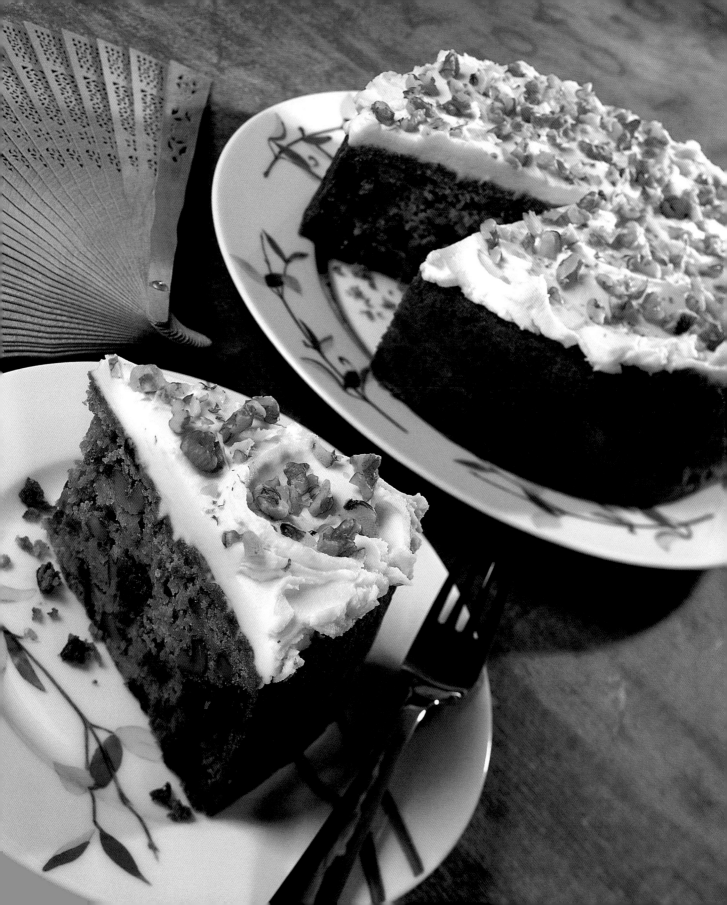

Date and *Gou Qi Zi* Chews

Dates are not only energising for spleen and stomach *Qi,* but will also nourish blood, so are ideal to eat in cases of anaemia. Combined with *Gou Qi Zi* (lycii berries) – especially helpful for liver and kidney – these chews make an energising, between-meals snack for tired men and women. They are also ideal for anaemia associated with menstrual bleeding.

Makes about 30-40 sweets

25g/1oz red dates (*Hong Zao*) – or use black dates (*Da Zao*) if red are not available
25g/1oz *Gou Qi Zi*
150g/5oz dried apricots (preferably organic)
115g/4oz dried figs (preferably organic)
25g/1oz raisins
1 piece of *Chen Pi* (tangerine peel)
150g/5oz butter
115g/4oz plain wholemeal flour
115g/4oz plain white flour
115g/4oz porridge oats or medium oatmeal
85g/3oz unrefined soft brown sugar

Preheat the oven to 200°C/400°F/gas mark 6. Thoroughly grease a shallow 28x18cm/11x7in cake tin.

Rinse the dates and *Gou Qi Zi* and soak in hot water for 10 minutes, then drain. Chop the dates, apricots and figs.

Put the dates, *Gou Qi Zi*, apricots, figs, raisins, *Chen Pi* and 6 tablespoons water in a saucepan and cook gently, stirring occasionally, until the mixture is soft.

Meanwhile, in a separate saucepan, melt the butter, then mix in the flours, oats or oatmeal and sugar.

Place half the oat mixture in the prepared cake tin and press down to level the surface. Cover with the dried fruit mixture. Spoon the remaining oat mixture over the top and press down firmly.

Bake in the oven for 20 minutes. Cool in the tin, then cut into small squares. Store in an airtight cake tin and eat as required.

A strong and efficient digestion is regarded in both Eastern and Western traditional medicine as essential to health.

The physicians of mediaeval Europe used to say that "death dwells in the bowels" suggesting that good digestion and diet were fundamental to health. This same emphasis is found in Chinese theory, where the *San Jiao* or triple burner epitomises the processes of digestion and healthy nutrition (see page 105). In the ancient Ayurvedic medicine of India, the digestive fire (*agni*) is regarded almost as a deity.

> Agni...*the digestive fire: the inner god: a being the size of our thumb dwells in the middle of our nature like a flame without smoke. He is the lord of what has been and what will be. He is yesterday and he is tomorrow.*
> *Katha Upanishad 2.12-13.*

Digestive imbalance is seen in a range of symptoms – from indigestion and constipation through to reduced immunity and low energy levels.

This section contains recipes that will not only strengthen overall digestive function, but will also help to combat imbalance and poor functionality. Many contain herbs which will strengthen spleen and stomach – the organs primarily associated with digestive function in Chinese theory – while others use more familiar Western culinary herbs which are often also effective digestive stimulants.

Strengthening the Digestion

Cranberries and *Yi Yi Ren* Soup

Like many cereals, *Yi Yi Ren* (Job's tears seed) is rich in nutrients, especially B vitamins and amino acids. When cooked, it has a soft mucilaginous texture which is easily digested, while helping to strengthen and soothe the system. It is a good tonic for the spleen, helps to ease symptoms of diarrhoea and is also diuretic, so will clear excess damp and regulate water metabolism. If you cannot find *Yi Yi Ren*, use pearl barley, which has similar nutritional, anti-diarrhoeal and soothing properties, although it is rather less diuretic.

Cranberries are rich in vitamin C and also help to soothe and cleanse the urinary tract. Recent studies have shown them to be an effective urinary antiseptic to ease cystitis and infections.

The Western herbs used in the dish are tonifying for the digestion, while the parsley is also diuretic.

Serves 4

1 onion, finely chopped
85g/3oz streaky bacon, diced
1 tablespoon olive oil
**225g/8oz *Yi Yi Ren* or pearl
    barley**
**1 potato, peeled and cut into
    1cm/½in cubes**
1 stick celery, thinly sliced
1 bay leaf
**115g/4oz fresh or frozen
    cranberries**
**1 tablespoon finely chopped
    fresh rosemary leaves**
**3 tablespoons finely chopped
    fresh parsley**
**6 finely chopped fresh basil
    leaves**
**4 finely chopped fresh sage
    leaves**
**Salt and freshly ground black
    pepper**

Sauté the onion and bacon in the oil in a large, thick-based saucepan for 3-4 minutes, until the onions have softened and the bacon is cooked.

Add the *Yi Yi Ren* or pearl barley, potato, celery and bay leaf and add enough water to cover the ingredients with 5cm/2in water to spare. Cover and simmer over a medium-low heat for about 1 hour, until the *Yi Yi Ren* is tender and the soup is thick, but adding more water if it becomes too thick.

After about 40-45 minutes, add the cranberries and 5 minutes before the end of the cooking time, add the rosemary.

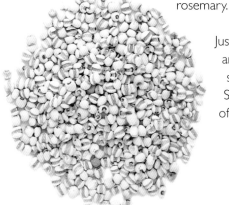

Just before serving, remove and discard the bay leaf, then stir in the remaining herbs. Season with salt and plenty of pepper.

Yi Yi Ren

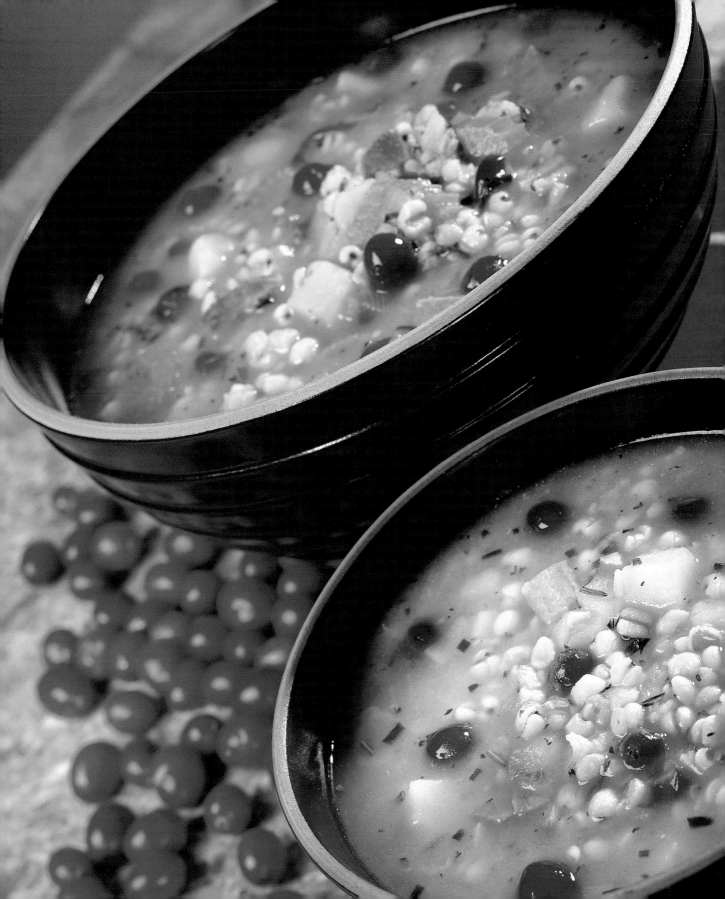

Forbidden Rice Salad

Forbidden rice (*Zi Mi*) is a black grain rice once cultivated for the sole use of China's Emperors as a health-giving food – it is now available in many Western supermarkets as well as Chinese stores. This sort of rice is highly nutritious with a nutty flavour and soft texture. Once cooked, the rice turns a deep purple colour.

In Chinese medicine, rice (*Mi*) is classified as sweet and neutral. As well as a staple food, rice is also eaten to ease many stomach and digestive problems including diarrhoea and indigestion.

Pink peppercorns are not a true pepper but are the almost ripe, soft berries of a South American tree *(Schinus terebinthifolius)*. They have no known therapeutic value but have a mild, sweet flavour ideal for vegetables, veal and game. They need to be used sparingly.

Serves 4

For the rice salad:
115g/4oz black rice
1 large onion, finely chopped
½ teaspoon salt
½ teaspoon coriander seeds
½ teaspoon paprika
1 green sweet pepper, deseeded and chopped
1 medium lettuce, shredded
2 tablespoons chopped fresh chives
2 tablespoons chopped fresh parsley or coriander

For the dressing:
1½ tablespoons basil oil (see Basics, page 188)
½ tablespoon chilli oil (see Basics, page 188)
1 tablespoon raspberry vinegar (see Basics, page 189)
Pinch of salt
1 teaspoon pink peppercorns

Rinse the black rice and place it in a saucepan with 225ml/8fl oz water. Add the onion, salt and spices and stir to mix. Bring to the boil, then cover, reduce the heat and simmer for 30 minutes. All the water should have been absorbed by this stage.

Mix all the dressing ingredients together thoroughly in a bowl or screw-top jar and pour over the warm rice. Cover the pan and allow the rice to stand until it is cold.

Combine the cooled rice with the green pepper and lettuce and garnish with chives and parsley or coriander.

Serve as a light lunch or with Asparagus Quiche (see page 22) or Thicky Herby Leek Tart (see page 169) for a more substantial meal.

Omelette with Morels

Morels (*Morchella esculenta*) are classified in Chinese medicine as sweet and cold. They are a valuable tonic for the stomach and digestion helping to reduce phlegm and normalise *Qi* flow.

Like other mushrooms, morels are rich in the essential amino acids needed to build protein so are helpful in debility and convalescence, as well as strengthening the digestion.

This omelette makes an ideal meal in convalescence or in digestive upsets.

Serves 1

25g/1oz dried morels or 85g/3oz fresh morels, sliced lengthwise

40g/1½oz butter

1 small shallot, chopped

Salt and freshly ground black pepper

2 eggs, beaten

2 tablespoons crème fraîche

Freshly grated Parmesan cheese, to garnish

Fresh morels have to be washed thoroughly under cold running water as the sponge-like caps often contain traces of earth. Trim the bases from the stems. Dried morels should be soaked in several changes of warm water for 15-20 minutes, then drained well.

Melt half the butter in a saucepan and sauté the morels and shallot for 3 minutes. Add salt and pepper to taste.

Meanwhile, beat together the eggs and crème fraîche with a little more salt and pepper to taste.

Melt the remaining butter in an omelette pan and pour in the egg mixture. Cook for a few minutes until the base is firm, then spoon the morels mixture over the top, fold over the omelette and serve garnished with Parmesan cheese.

Fennel and Celery Soup

Fennel has been used since ancient times as a digestive remedy – extracts of the seeds are still used in baby's gripe water to combat colic. Celery seeds, too, are an important medicinal herb helping to clear uric acid from arthritic joints and acting as a diuretic – especially useful for fluid retention in pre-menstrual syndrome (PMS).

This soup uses the stems and leaves rather than the seeds, so it has a milder action as a warming digestive remedy, ideal for those suffering from stomach chills or weak digestion. It also makes a comforting food for those suffering from PMS.

If you like the flavour of fennel and celery seeds, then add a teaspoon of seeds of each plant to enhance the dish's therapeutic effect.

Serves 4

15g/½oz butter
2 onions, chopped
1 fennel bulb, thinly sliced
3 sticks celery, thinly sliced
1 litre/1¾ pints chicken or vegetable stock
2 tablespoons sour cream
115g/4oz smoked ham or cooked bacon, cut into thin strips (optional)
Salt and freshly ground black pepper
1-2 tablespoons chopped fresh dill

Melt the butter in a large saucepan and sauté the onions, fennel and celery for 4-5 minutes.

Add the stock, bring to the boil, cover and simmer for about 15-20 minutes until the vegetables are tender.

Add the sour cream and reheat the soup, taking care that it does not boil and curdle. Stir in the ham or bacon strips, then add salt and pepper to taste.

Serve sprinkled with a little chopped dill.

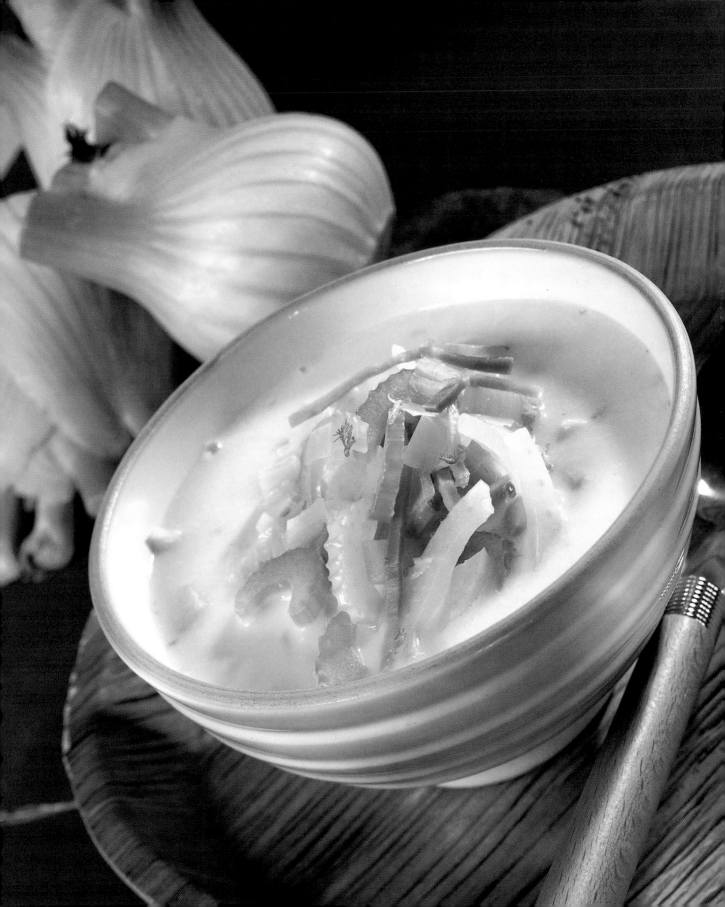

Prawns and Papaya

Papaya fruits are regarded as a traditional remedy for digestive upsets in many parts of the East. The fruit is now known to contain an enzyme called papain which actually helps to improve the digestion of certain chemicals, so making the system more efficient.

Papaya is ideal added to fruit salads or is delicious – as here – combined with large prawns and honey, which also helps the digestion.

Serves 4 as a starter or 2 for lunch

For the sauce:
Juice of 2 limes
4 tablespoons walnut oil
1 teaspoon Dijon mustard
1 teaspoon clear honey
Salt and freshly ground black pepper

For the prawns and papaya:
1 large ripe papaya
12 cooked king prawns, peeled and with heads removed
Coriander or flat-leaf parsley leaves, to garnish

Make the sauce by whisking all the ingredients together thoroughly. Set aside.

Peel the papaya, cut in half and scoop out the seeds. Slice the flesh into 12 segments.

Arrange 3 prawns and 3 papaya segments on each plate and divide the sauce between the plates. Garnish with the parsley or coriander leaves and serve.

Rice Porridge with *Yi Yi Ren* and *Bian Dou*

This porridge is especially useful for those suffering from weak, sluggish digestion. It can be served as a light supper dish or lunch – although the Chinese would also eat similar porridges for breakfast.

The kidney beans are high in protein while the *Yi Yi Ren* (Job's tears seeds) and *Bian Dou* (hyacinth beans) both help to strengthen the spleen and remove excess damp and phlegm. The spring onions (*Cong Bai*) are also therapeutic – helping to disperse cold, strengthen *Qi* and warm the stomach.

The porridge is ideal for acute illnesses or fevers involving gastric upsets.

Serves 6

25g/1oz red kidney beans (canned or fresh)

4oz round grain rice

15g/½oz *Yi Yi Ren*

15g/½oz *Bian Dou*

1 litre/1¾ pints water or vegetable stock

Bunch of spring onions, chopped, to garnish

If using fresh kidney beans, wash, cover with water and leave to soak overnight. Drain, rinse and cover with fresh water, then bring to the boil and boil vigorously for 45-50 minutes before straining. If using canned beans, drain them well.

Add the rice, *Yi Yi Ren*, *Bian Dou* and water or stock to the cooked kidney beans in a large saucepan, bring to the boil and simmer for 45-60 minutes, until the rice is cooked. Add more water or stock during cooking if necessary, to prevent the mixture becoming dry. The rice grains will absorb most of the water and burst to produce a thick porridge.

Serve in soup bowls and garnish with spring onions.

Hearty Fish Soup with *Lian Ou, Chen Pi* and Chinese Dates

This soup is ideal both for strengthening the digestion and replenishing *Qi* and blood. If you want a soup that is more nourishing for the blood, use *Hong Zao* (red dates) instead of *Da Zao* (black dates) and add a handful of *Gou Qi Zi* (lycii berries) in the last 30 minutes of cooking. It is then ideal as an energising food for all ages, and especially suitable for women suffering from menstrual problems or iron-deficient anaemia.

Lotus root (*Lian Ou* or *Lian Gen*) is cold with a sweet flavour. When cooked, it helps to strengthen the spleen, aids the digestion and replenishes blood. It is a useful food for poorly healing tissues. Cooked lotus roots have a crunchy flavour and are often added to Chinese soups.

Serves 4-6

1 fresh *Lian Ou* (or pre-cooked canned lotus root)
1kg/2¼lb mixed fresh fish (cleaned, left on the bone)
2 onions, chopped
1 leek, thinly sliced
2.5cm/1in slice fresh root ginger, peeled and finely chopped
3 cloves garlic, sliced
1 tablespoon olive oil
2 carrots, diced
2 sticks celery, sliced
6 fresh shiitake mushrooms
450g/1lb tomatoes, skinned, deseeded and chopped (or 400g/14oz can organic chopped tomatoes)
1 bay leaf
6 black dates (*Da Zao*)
2-3 pieces *Chen Pi*
Juice of 1 orange
Chopped parsley, to garnish

If using fresh *Lian Ou*, peel and slice the root diagonally and place in a saucepan. Cover with 570ml/1 pint water, bring to the boil and simmer, covered, for 2 hours.

Wash the fish – red mullet or monkfish are ideal for this recipe – and cut into thick pieces, cutting through the bone. Set aside.

Sauté the onion, leek, ginger and garlic in the oil in a large saucepan over a very gentle heat for 10 minutes. Do not brown.

Add the carrots, celery and sliced shiitake mushrooms to the pan and cook until soft. Add the tomatoes and bay leaf and simmer gently for 10 minutes over a low heat to produce plenty of juice. Add the Chinese dates, *Chen Pi* and orange juice and stir to mix.

Add enough water to the cooked *Lian Ou* and its cooking water (or canned lotus root) to bring the volume back up to 570ml/1 pint and add this to the soup mixture. Bring to the boil and simmer for 20 minutes.

Add the chunks of fish and simmer for a further 10-12 minutes, until the fish is cooked and tender.

Garnish with the parsley and serve with fresh bread.

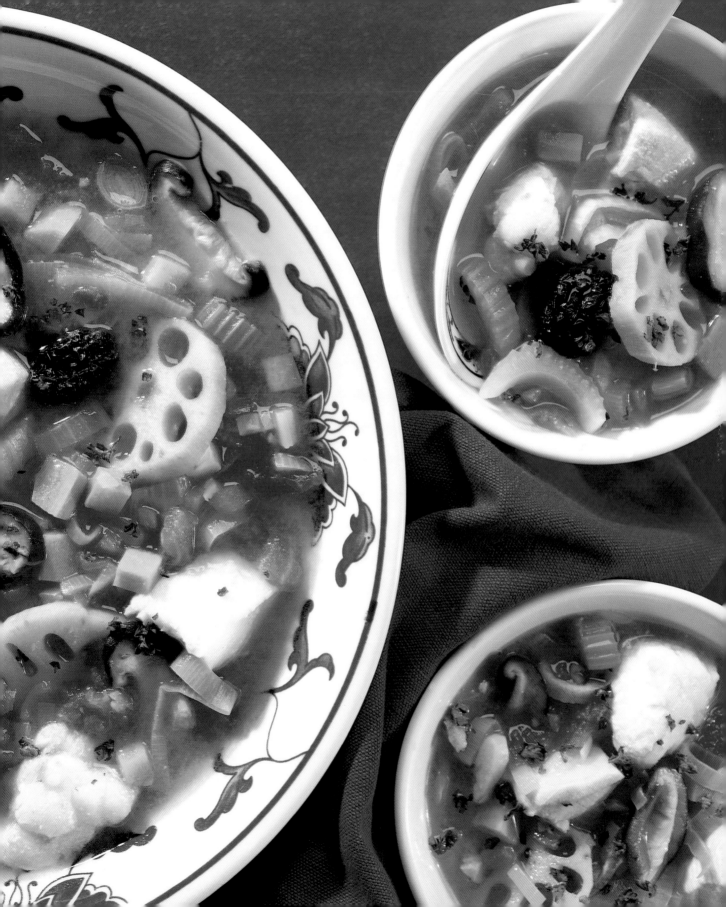

All Sorts of Mashed Potatoes

Potatoes are rather more than a simple staple providing filling carbohydrates for hungry eaters. They are an important source of vitamin C, rich in B-complex vitamins (including B_1, B_5, B_6 and folic acid) and containing several essential minerals including iron, calcium, manganese, magnesium and phosphorus.

Potato juice is used therapeutically to relieve digestive problems associated with excessive stomach acid – including indigestion, gastritis and peptic ulcers – and it is a good liver remedy which can also be helpful for bile stones and gall bladder problems.

Potatoes can also provide a suitable base for additional healing remedies – as in these suggestions.

Serves 4
Basic mashed potato:
8 medium potatoes, peeled and cut into halves or quarters
Pinch of salt
2 tablespoons milk
15g/½oz butter

Put the potatoes into a pan of cold water with a pinch of salt, bring to the boil and simmer for 15-20 minutes (cooking time will depend on the size and age of the potatoes) or until the potatoes are soft. Drain and mash the potatoes, adding the butter and milk and mixing well.

Anchovy Mash

Anchovies are classified as warm, sweet and *yang* – ideal to combat problems associated with excess fluids and cold. Add 6-8 anchovy fillets, very finely chopped, to the mashed potatoes to help balance cooler fish dishes in winter or as an additional energy boost.

Herby Mash

Oregano and thyme are stimulating, warming herbs which are both carminative to ease digestive upsets. Add 1 tablespoon finely chopped fresh oregano and 2 teaspoons finely chopped fresh thyme to the mashed potatoes and serve with roast or fatty meats to help the digestion.

Sesame Mash

Sesame is stimulating for the stomach and lower bowel, helping to encourage digestive function and lubricating dryness. Instead of the butter, mash the potatoes with 2 tablespoons sour cream and sprinkle 25g/1oz toasted sesame seeds over the top before serving. Alternatively, replace the butter with 1 tablespoon sesame seed oil.

Roast Salmon with Pesto

Salmon is an energising fish which expels cold, warms the stomach and harmonises the middle *Jiao*. It can be helpful for general digestive weakness and is a good food in debility and convalescence.

The triple burner or *San Jiao*, is an attempt, dating back to 2500BC, to represent the body's digestive function in some way. It is sometimes described as a formless sewage system which transports and transforms nutrients while eliminating waste material. It can be a difficult concept for Westerners and is perhaps best regarded as a generalisation of internal functions related to water regulation and digestion. It has three components – upper, middle and lower *Jiao* – with the middle *Jiao* between diaphragm and navel, closely linked to the functions of spleen and stomach.

In this dish, salmon is combined with pesto – you can either use coriander pesto, which is a good detoxifier, helping to clear heavy metals from the system (see page 120) or make the same sauce using basil instead. Basil is hot and pungent and helps reduce dampness and phlegm. Although culinary sweet basil (*Ocimum basilicum*) may lack the potent spiritual powers attributed to holy basil (see page 72), it is still uplifting, energising and anti-depressant, while rocket helps stimulate the liver.

Serves 4

5 cloves garlic, peeled but left whole

3 tablespoons extra-virgin olive oil

4 salmon fillets, each about 150-175g/5-6oz, with skin still attached: ideally use thick square pieces rather than long thin ones

Seasoned plain flour, for coating

3-4 tablespoons pesto

Fresh basil or rocket leaves, shredded, to garnish

Preheat the oven to 200°C/400°F/gas mark 6. Put the whole garlic cloves into a roasting tin with the olive oil and bake in the oven for 15 minutes.

Descale the salmon fillets and coat with seasoned flour. Transfer the roasting dish to the hob and cook the salmon, skin side down, for 2 minutes.

Increase the oven temperature to 240°C/475°F/gas mark 9. Turn the salmon fillets skin side up and return the dish to the oven for 3 minutes.

Serve the salmon fillets on individual plates with mashed potatoes and a spoonful of the pesto. Garnish with the shredded herb leaves.

Chicken with Tarragon Mustard

Chicken is a warm, sweet meat which is especially beneficial for spleen and stomach. It helps tonify *Jing* (essence), so is an ideal food for the elderly. It also helps energise *Qi* and blood and is warming for the middle *Jiao* – closely associated with the energy of digestion (see page 105).

It is combined here with tarragon *(Artemisia dracunculus),* which is usually regarded as purely a culinary flavouring but is also a good digestive tonic – bitter and aromatic. Additionally, it has a stimulating effect on the womb, so this dish would also be helpful for menstrual problems. Tarragon is also diuretic – serving the dish with steamed asparagus would make it additionally beneficial for fluid retention associated with premenstrual syndrome.

Serves 4

4 skinless, boneless chicken breasts, each about 115g/4oz in weight

2 tablespoons extra-virgin olive oil

1 tablespoon tarragon mustard (see Basics, page 187)

120ml/4fl oz dry white wine

150ml/¼ pint chicken stock (optional)

200g/7oz crème fraîche

Salt and freshly ground black pepper

Cut each chicken breast through lengthwise to make 3 long chunky strips. Heat the oil in a frying pan or wok and sauté the chicken strips for 7-8 minutes until they are well browned and the chicken juices run clear when tested with a skewer. Transfer the chicken pieces to a serving dish and keep warm.

Add the mustard and wine to the pan or wok, stir to blend with the cooking juices and bubble for 2-3 minutes to evaporate the alcohol. If you prefer a more liquid sauce, add the stock and simmer for 3-4 minutes until well blended with the mustard mixture.

Lower the heat to a gentle simmer and add the crème fraîche. Stir to give a smooth well-mixed sauce and then return the chicken pieces to the pan. Simmer for 2-3 minutes to heat through, then season to taste with salt and pepper. Serve with plain boiled rice.

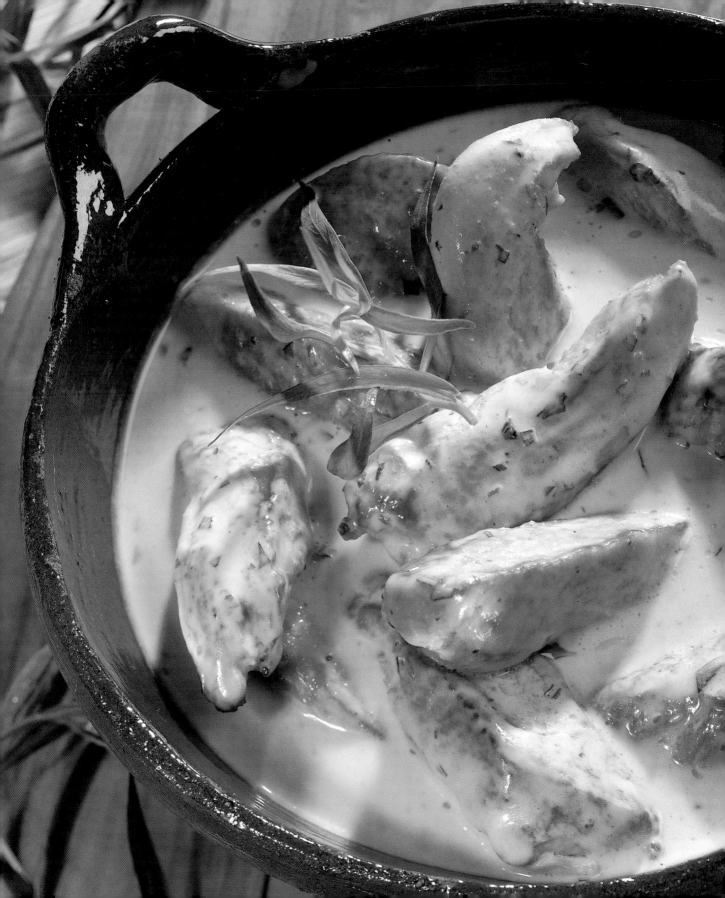

Savoury *Fu Ling* Dumplings

Fu Ling (known in the West as Indian bread or tuckahoe) is a solid fungus which grows on the roots of fir trees. It is an important Chinese medicinal herb used to strengthen the digestion and is good for those with sluggish damp digestions, helping to relieve abdominal bloating, water retention and diarrhoea. *Fu Ling* also nourishes the heart, calms the spirit and helps insomnia and nervousness.

These dumplings are an ideal general tonic, especially suitable for those with weak digestions.

Serves 5-10

6 water chestnuts, fresh or canned
2 medium Jerusalem artichokes
115g/4oz minced pork
115g/4oz peeled prawns
115g/4oz shiitake mushrooms
1 tablespoon shoyu soy sauce
1 tablespoon sesame oil
55g/2oz powdered *Fu Ling*
30 wonton wrappers (buy fresh or frozen from a Chinese supermarket)

Peel the water chestnuts (if fresh) and the Jerusalem artichokes, then blend in a blender or food processor with the pork, prawns, shiitake mushrooms, shoyu, sesame oil and *Fu Ling* to make a paste.

Place a small amount of the paste in the centre of each wonton wrapper, wet the edges of the wrappers with water and pinch together to shape into a bundle.

Place the dumplings in a bamboo steamer on greaseproof or non-stick baking paper and steam for 8-10 minutes until cooked.

Serve with a little more shoyu as a starter or as part of a Chinese meal.

Mushroom Sauce with Pasta

Common button mushrooms *(Agaricus bisporus)* are characterised in Chinese theory as cool and sweet, acting on the large intestine, stomach, spleen and lungs. As well as a common folk remedy for diarrhoea and nausea, they are also an ingredient in traditional "tendon-easing-powder" used in China to ease numbed limbs and discomfort in tendons and veins.

Tomatoes, among their many other attributes, also strengthen the stomach and encourage digestive function and they are a common remedy for poor appetite or weight loss.

The Western herbs in this recipe also help to ease digestion and stimulate the appetite.

Serves 4

1 small sprig of fresh thyme, finely chopped
1 sprig of fresh marjoram, finely chopped
6-8 large basil leaves, finely chopped
2 tablespoons dry Martini
1 onion, chopped
1-2 leeks, washed and thinly sliced
2-3 cloves garlic, crushed
2 tablespoons plus 1 teaspoon olive oil
225g/8oz button mushrooms
8 tomatoes, skinned and chopped
Salt and freshly ground black pepper
2 tablespoons single or double cream (optional)
280g/10oz spaghetti
Grated Parmesan cheese, to garnish (optional)

First make the sauce. Put the thyme, marjoram and basil in a dish and cover with dry Martini. Cover and set aside. This could be done a few hours or even a day in advance.

Fry the onion, leek and garlic in 2 tablespoons oil. Add the mushrooms and tomatoes, bring to the boil and simmer for 15 minutes.

Add the herbs and Martini mix and simmer for a further 5 minutes. Season to taste with salt and pepper, stir in the cream, if using, and then remove the pan from the heat.

Meanwhile, cook the pasta as directed on the pack, in a saucepan of lightly salted, boiling water with the remaining 1 teaspoon oil added. until it is *al dente*.

Drain the pasta, transfer it to a serving dish and pour over the vegetable sauce. Serve with a green salad. If the cream is omitted, garnish with grated Parmesan cheese.

Sweet Potato and *Chen Pi* Cakes

Sweet potatoes are warm with a sweet flavour. They tonify *yang, Qi* and blood and are especially beneficial for spleen and kidneys. Combined with black sesame seeds, they help lubricate and move the bowels so act as a gentle stimulant for a sluggish digestion.

Chen Pi (tangerine peel) is a rich source of vitamin C and aids digestion of these sweet cakes. It is traditionally used to combat indigestion and nausea and also helps to tonify spleen *Qi*. If you cannot find *Chen Pi*, dry your own organic, unwaxed tangerine peel and use that instead.

Makes about 25

10g/⅓oz *Chen Pi*
3 sweet potatoes, each about 200g/7oz to yield 350g/ 12oz mashed potatoes
2 eggs, plus 1 egg white
350g/12oz unrefined caster sugar
25g/1oz unsalted butter
150g/5oz ground almonds
1 tablespoon lime or lemon juice
1-2 tablespoons black sesame seeds

Preheat the oven to 200°C/400°F/gas mark 6. Cover the *Chen Pi* with boiling water and leave to soak for 15-20 minutes. Drain and chop the softened *Chen Pi* finely, then set aside.

To prepare the sweet potatoes, bake them in their skins in the oven for 40-60 minutes, depending on their size, until they are cooked and tender. Remove from the oven and reduce the oven temperature to 190°C/375°F/gas mark 5.

When the potatoes are cool enough to handle, peel and discard the skin and mash the flesh. Beat the whole eggs, sugar and butter together. Place the mixture in a saucepan and stir in the almonds, sweet potato mash, lemon or lime juice and chopped *Chen Pi*. Beat together until well mixed.

Heat the mixture over a low heat and stir continuously for 10 minutes or until it thickens to the consistency of stiff mashed potato, making sure that the mixture does not stick to the pan.

Turn out onto a floured surface or board, spread out evenly and leave to cool slightly. When cool enough to handle, take plum-sized pieces of mixture with floured hands and mould into 5cm/2in round cakes. Place all the cakes on greaseproof paper on a baking tray. Brush with a little beaten egg white and sprinkle with black sesame seeds.

Bake in the oven for 20 minutes. Serve cool.

Black sesame seeds

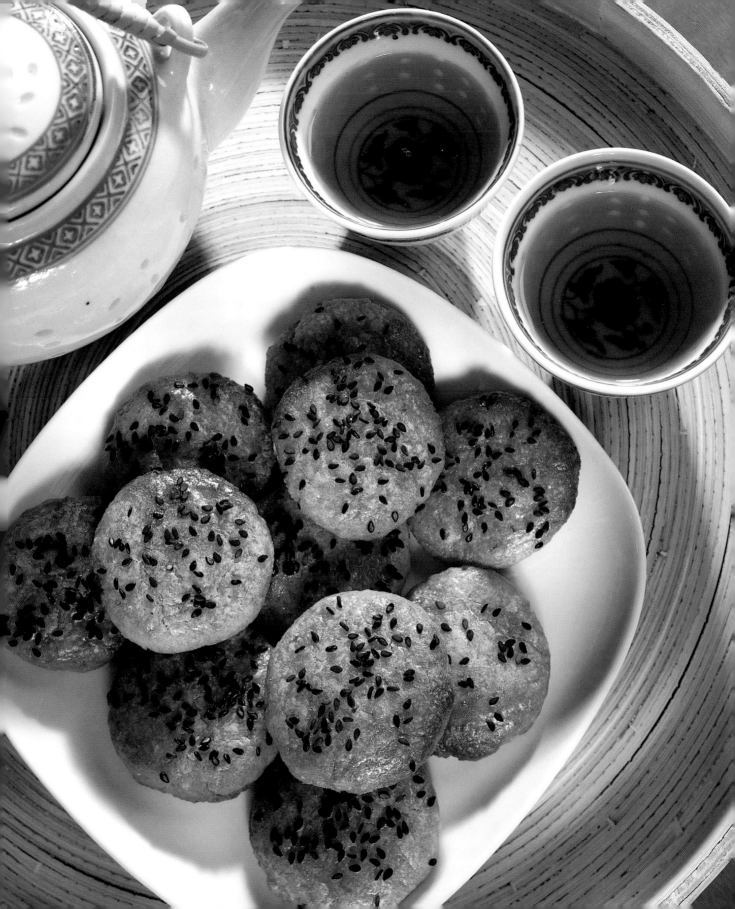

Milk Custard with Ginger

Milk custard always makes a soothing and easily-digestible food for upset stomachs and digestive disorders. Add ginger and you have a warming remedy that will also combat nausea and vomiting – it's ideal for children prone to bilious attacks as well as for adults with gastritis or general digestive weakness.

Serves 4

- **1 thick large thumb-size piece fresh root ginger, peeled**
- **700ml/1¼ pints cow's milk or soya milk**
- **3 tablespoons granulated sugar**
- **2 egg whites**

Purée the ginger in a blender or food processor until it is smooth, then spoon it into a clean muslin cloth and squeeze tightly to release the ginger juice. Discard the ginger pulp.

In a bowl, whisk together the milk, sugar, egg whites and ginger juice and pour into four rice bowls. Steam the custards in a lidded steamer over a pan of boiling water or use a bamboo steamer in a wok. Be careful to keep the water at a gentle simmer only, so that the custard remains smooth. It will take about 20 minutes to set. Serve warm.

Mint and Raspberry Sauce

Mint (*Mentha* x *piperita*) leaves are cooling and good for clearing common colds associated with external "wind-heat evils", as well as helping with the digestion of rich foods. Mint also helps regulate menstruation, calms mood swings and eases abdominal distension.

Raspberries are neutral with a sweet flavour. They are tonifying to the liver and kidneys, helping to strengthen the eyesight and ease problems of impotence and excessive urination associated with deficient kidney *yang*.

This aromatic sauce is not only good to eat – it is especially suitable for menstrual disorders, in old age or exhaustion, and to stimulate a weakened digestion.

Serves 8

- **280g/10oz fresh raspberries**
- **85g/3oz caster sugar**
- **2 tablespoons lime juice**
- **1 sprig of fresh mint, plus 10 fresh mint leaves**

Place the raspberries, sugar, lime juice, sprig of mint and 4 tablespoons water in a saucepan and gently dissolve the sugar over a low heat, stirring all the time. Bring gently to the boil, then simmer for 10 minutes.

Remove and discard the mint sprig and finely chop the mint leaves. Stir the chopped mint into the sauce and pour over fruit salad or onto Greek yoghurt in individual bowls.

Bilberry Cheesecake

Bilberries may seem no more than a traditional topping for cheesecakes but the combination is very astringent and drying – ideal for diarrhoea or digestive upsets associated with damp and phlegm. The bilberries contain a blue pigment (myrtillin) which has an affinity for bacteria cells, entering and damaging them. The effect is not enough to kill the bacteria but it has been shown to inhibit their growth, so bilberries are an ideal food for any sort of gastric infection as well.

Soft cheeses have a similar anti-diarrhoeal effect so the traditional bilberry-topped cheesecake makes an ideal food during attacks of summer diarrhoea or when recovering from food poisoning. Ideally, the bilberries should be unsweetened, but they tend to be quite sour and not to everyone's taste.

Serves 6-8

8 digestive biscuits, crushed
450g/1lb curd cheese
175g/6oz sour cream
2 eggs
25g/1oz softened butter
115g/4oz granulated sugar
225g/8oz bilberries
25g/1oz caster sugar
1-2 teaspoons arrowroot
Icing sugar, whipped cream
 or crème fraîche, to serve
 (optional)

Preheat the oven to 190°C/375°F/gas mark 5. Spread the crushed biscuits evenly across the bottom of a greased 20cm/8in flan dish. Mix the curd cheese, sour cream, eggs, butter and granulated sugar together until smooth, then spoon evenly over the crushed biscuits.

Bake in the centre of the oven for 10 minutes, then reduce the oven temperature to 170°C/325°F/gas mark 3 and bake for a further 30 minutes or until the cheesecake is firm and golden yellow – a skewer inserted into the centre should come out clean. Remove the cheesecake from the oven and allow it to cool.

Meanwhile, gently simmer the bilberries, caster sugar and 3-4 tablespoons water together in a pan for 15-20 minutes or until the berries are soft. Rub the mixture through a sieve or blend in a blender or food processor to make a smooth purée.

Return the purée to the pan and reheat until simmering. Mix the arrowroot with a little water to make a paste and then stir into the bilberry purée. Cook for 4-5 minutes, stirring, until the mixture starts to thicken. Remove the pan from the heat and set aside to cool.

Once cool, spoon the bilberry topping over the cooled cheesecake. If you really must sweeten the bilberries further, sprinkle with a layer of sifted icing sugar and serve the cheesecake with whipped cream or crème fraîche.

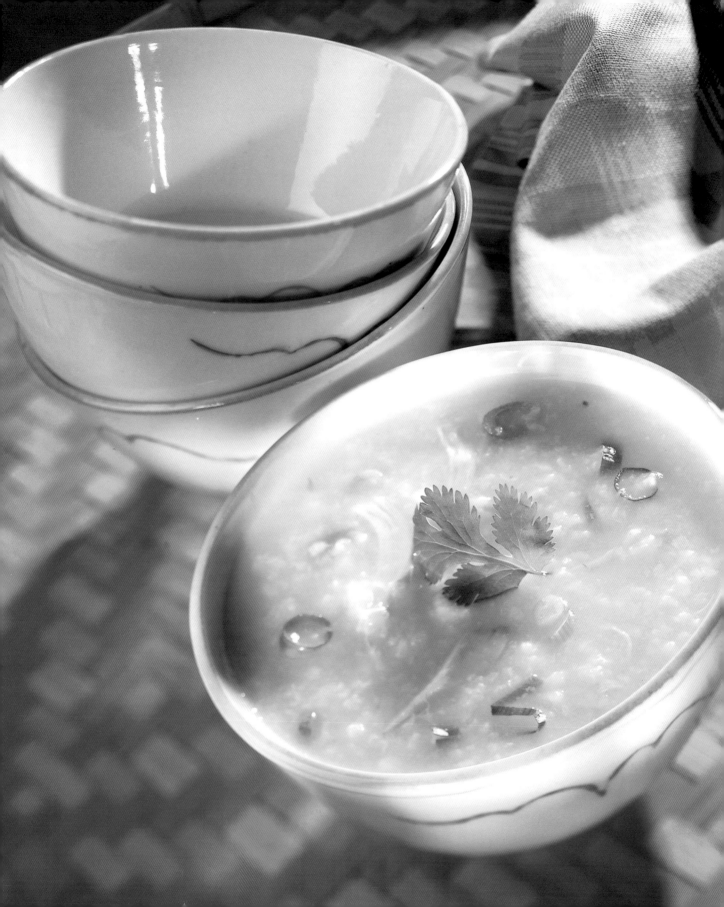

Soothing foods that are comforting and easy to digest are ideal when recovering from illness or exhaustion. The system is often too weak for strongly energising foods containing powerful tonic herbs and the body needs bland tastes and gentle stimulation.

Illness is often associated with a build up of toxins in the system – difficult to digest chemicals clogging the liver and joints made worse by the many pollutants encountered in Western society.

Chinese families will make a variety of therapeutic rice dishes for treating minor household ills, when recovering from illness or to support prescribed herbal remedies. They're usually called *congee* by Westerners after the Anglo-Indian word for porridge, although the Chinese refer to these remedies as *Shi-fan* or water rice.

Congees have been recommended for a range of ailments since ancient times. In Buddhist tradition, congee made with milk and honey was regarded as a general preventative for ill health. It was said to confer "life and beauty, ease and strength", and would dispel "hunger, thirst and wind", as well as helping digestion and "cleansing the bladder".

Cleanse and Comfort: foods for convalescents and to detoxify

Basic Chicken Congee (recipe on page 116)

Basic Chicken Congee

Congee is traditionally made by putting a cup of rice with 6 cups of water in a heavy-based, covered saucepan. The pot is set on the lowest possible heat on the hob and simmered for up to 6 hours, stirring regularly to prevent the congee from sticking.

Plain congee is often served for breakfast in parts of China with an assortment of side dishes, such as hard-boiled eggs or steamed buns. Additional ingredients can also be added to the rice mix to create a variety of therapeutic meals.

This Western version of a basic chicken congee is easy to make and digest. It is soothing and nourishing for both the young and old and is ideal for convalescents, those suffering from exhaustion or over-work, or when recovering from gastric upsets.

Serves 4-6

1 medium, free range chicken (skin removed), about 1.5kg/3½lb

200g/7oz long grain white or brown rice

5cm/2in piece fresh root ginger, peeled and grated

1 teaspoon soy sauce

1 teaspoon sesame seed oil

Pinch of sea salt and freshly ground black pepper

1 bunch spring onions, finely chopped

Chopped fresh coriander leaves, to garnish

Put the chicken, rice and ginger into a large saucepan. Cover with water and bring to the boil. Reduce the heat, cover and simmer gently for 2-3 hours or until the chicken is falling off the bones and the rice is soft. Add more water if necessary during cooking to prevent the congee from boiling dry.

Remove the pan from the heat, remove and discard the chicken carcass and bones, then shred the chicken and return it to the congee.

Stir in the soy sauce, sesame seed oil and salt and pepper. Serve in soup bowls, garnished with chopped spring onions and coriander.

The herbalist Li Shi Zhen recommended a variety of congees in his great herbal, the *Ben Cao Gang Mu*, written between 1552 and 1578. Among his additions to a basic rice congee were:

- ginger congee – adding dried ginger to the mix to combat "cold and deficiency" problems that may lead to indigestion and diarrhoea;
- liver congee – with chopped liver added to the mixture as a remedy for "liver deficiency syndromes";
- aduki bean congee – to help with fluid retention and urinary dysfunction;
- leek or onion congee – as a warming remedy for the digestive system, suitable for treating diarrhoea.

You can vary the basic chicken congee with these additional herbs and foods to suit particular needs.

Spiced Winter Lamb

This dish boosts *Qi* and is ideal as a general energy tonic or in debility and convalescence. The combination of lamb and herbs especially strengthens kidney *yin, yang* and *Qi*, while the warming herbs – ginger, cinnamon and ginseng – are moderated by *Yu Zhu* (Solomon's seal), which is more cooling. *Yu Zhu* also nourishes *yin* and will ease muscular pains.

The squash is warming and sweet to strengthen the digestion as do the Chinese dates which also tonify *Qi* and blood.

Serves 4-6

5 *Hong Zao* (red dates)
5 *Da Zao* (black dates)
10g/⅓oz or 3 pieces of *Chen Pi*
  (tangerine peel)
10g/⅓oz *Yu Zhu*
10g/⅓oz ginseng or *Dang Shen*
3 cloves garlic, crushed
1 thumb-sized piece fresh
  root ginger, peeled and
  finely chopped or minced
1 teaspoon ground coriander
Juice of 1 lemon
1.2kg/2¾lb shoulder of lamb
1 teaspoon ground ginger
½ teaspoon *Rou Gui* (ground
  cinnamon)
1 bunch coriander, stalks and
  leaves chopped separately
115g/4oz organic dried
  apricots
3 sweet peppers – 1 each of
  orange/yellow, red and
  green, deseeded and diced
500g/1lb 2oz butternut
  squash, peeled, deseeded
  and diced
300g/10½oz couscous
1 tablespoon walnut oil

Soak the dates, *Chen Pi, Yu Zhu* and ginseng or *Dang Shen* in 850ml/1½ pints water and leave for at least 2 hours, or overnight. Bring to the boil and simmer for 40 minutes.

Meanwhile, combine the garlic, root ginger, ground coriander and lemon juice and pour over the lamb. Leave to marinate for 2-3 hours in a cool place or overnight in the refrigerator.

Preheat the oven to 180°C/350°F/gas mark 4. Place the lamb in a roasting dish and cook for 45 minutes per kg or 20 minutes per lb plus 20 minutes, until the juices run clear (total cooking time is about 1¼ hours). Discard the marinade.

While the lamb is roasting add the ground ginger, *Rou Gui*, chopped coriander stalks, apricots, sweet peppers and squash to the herbal decoction and bring to the boil. Cover and simmer over a medium heat for 15 minutes or until the vegetables are cooked.

Strain the vegetable mixture over a measuring jug and keep warm; discard the *Chen Pi*. Make up the strained cooking liquid to 400ml/14fl oz with boiling water if necesssary.

Mix the couscous with the walnut oil and then pour the hot cooking liquid over the couscous. Stir to mix and leave to stand for 10 minutes.

Serve the couscous topped with the vegetable mixture and chopped coriander leaves alongside the carved roast lamb.

Beetroot Salad with Onion and Horseradish

Beetroot is nutritious and energising, rich in potassium, silica, iron, amino acids and vitamins A, B, and C. It is ideal as a blood tonic in anaemia and is traditionally used in debilitating diseases and convalescence. It is neutral with a sweet taste and acts as a tonic for *Qi*, blood and *yin*. Horse-radish is stimulating, pungent, sweet and hot to energise *yang* and clear damp and phlegm. It clears food stagnation and phlegm-heat from the lungs. Onion, like garlic, is a good anti-bacterial. This salad makes an energising lunch or starter which is also ideal during colds, flu and convalescence.

Serves 3-4

300g/10oz cooked beetroot
1 tablespoon horseradish
1 onion, finely chopped
2-3 tablespoons olive oil
1-2 tablespoons wine or
　cider vinegar
Salt and black pepper
2 tablespoons chopped
　fresh parsley, to garnish

Grate the peeled beetroot into a bowl and mix with the grated fresh horseradish and onion.

To make the dressing, combine the olive oil, vinegar and salt and pepper and mix well.

Pour the dressing over the beetroot mixture and toss to mix. Garnish with the chopped parsley. Serve with crisp French bread for a light lunch or starter, or with Thick Herby Leek Tart (see page 169) for a more substantial meal.

Fast Beetroot Soup

Beef stock helps provide vital amino acids and nutrients for strengthening muscles and bones, making this soup an ideal remedy for those recovering from illness. The thyme, as well as adding flavour, is highly anti-bacterial to help combat lingering infection.

Serves 4-6

3 tablespoons olive oil
3 medium beetroots, grated
1 large carrot, grated
1 onion, finely chopped
1 leek, cut into thin strips
1 clove garlic, crushed
1 litre/1¾ pints beef stock
2-3 teaspoons fresh thyme
Salt and black pepper
2 tablespoons natural yoghurt

Heat the oil in a saucepan and fry the vegetables and garlic for 2-3 minutes.

Add the stock, bring to the boil, cover and simmer for about 20 minutes or until the vegetables are soft. Add the thyme 5 minutes before the end of the cooking time, with salt and pepper to taste.

Remove the pan from the heat and stir in the yoghurt just before serving.

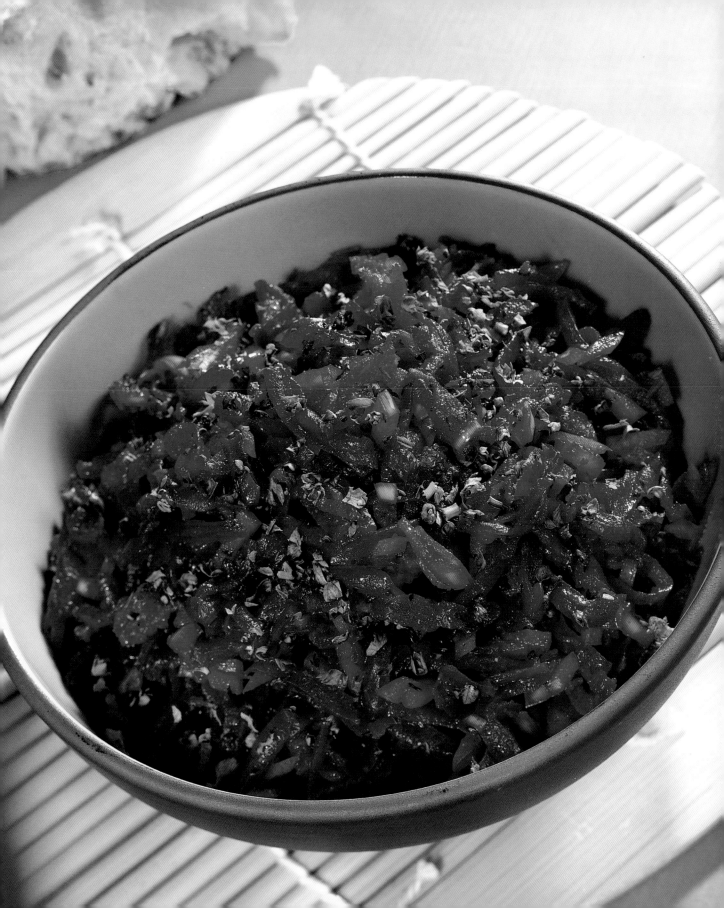

Fresh Coriander Leaf Pesto with Pasta

Best known from its use in Indian and Middle Eastern cookery, coriander has become a familiar culinary herb over the past few years with a characteristic earthy flavour. Coriander seeds are a valuable medicinal herb traditionally used for minor digestive problems.

According to recent Japanese research, coriander leaves can accelerate the excretion of toxic metals such as mercury, lead and aluminium from the body. Unless they are removed by chemicals called "chelating agents", these heavy metals remain in the body forever, with high levels now blamed for certain arthritic conditions, depression, memory loss, muscle pain and weakness.

Eating plenty of coriander is thus an inexpensive and easy way to remove (or "chelate") toxic metals from the nervous system and body tissue. People suffering from the ill effects of mercury amalgam dental fillings, would benefit from eating coriander. It can be added raw to soups or salads or used as a garnish with practically any savoury dish.

Coriander leaves are fine and feathery and almost disappear once the flowers arrive, but a leafy cultivar (cilantro) is now more readily available and is well worth growing in the herb garden – it also makes an excellent substitute for basil in pesto sauce.

Serves 4

I handful of fresh, organically grown coriander leaves, washed
6 tablespoons olive oil
I clove garlic, peeled
2 tablespoons lightly roasted almonds
2 tablespoons lemon juice
225g/8oz fresh pasta such as spaghetti or tagliatelle
Salt
55g/2oz crumbled feta cheese
Grated Parmesan cheese and freshly ground black pepper, to garnish

Put the coriander and olive oil in a blender or food processor and blend until finely chopped. Add all the remaining ingredients except the pasta, feta cheese, salt and garnish, and process to form a lumpy paste. You can alter the consistency by changing the amount of olive oil and lemon juice, but keep the 3:1 ratio of oil to juice.

Cook the pasta in a pan of lightly salted, boiling water, as directed on the pack, then drain well and spoon over the pesto immediately so that it melts into the hot pasta.

Add the feta cheese, toss well and sprinkle generously with grated Parmesan and freshly ground black pepper to garnish. Serve immediately.

The pesto freezes well, so make several batches at once during the coriander season and freeze in small containers.

Pasta Ring with Coriander Pesto Chicken

This is a good way of using the coriander pesto in the last recipe for a main meal. Chicken is warming for stomach and spleen, and helps to regulate digestion so will also play a part in cleansing the system.

Serves 6

For the pasta ring:
1 teaspoon salt
450g/1lb thin ribbon pasta,
   mixed colours if possible
2 pimientos, thinly sliced
6 skinless, boneless chicken
   breasts, each about
   115g/4oz
1 tablespoon olive oil
1 quantity coriander pesto
   (see opposite)

For the dressing:
2 teaspoons garlic oil
2 teaspoons basil oil
2 teaspoons raspberry
   vinegar
2 teaspoons orange peel
   vinegar
Salt and freshly ground
   black pepper

3-4 sprigs of fresh
   coriander, to garnish

Bring a large pan of water to the boil and add 1 teaspoon salt. Cook the pasta in the water until it is *al dente* (approximately 6-12 minutes depending on the type of pasta used). Drain in a colander and rinse with boiling water.

Make the dressing by whisking all the dressing ingredients together until well mixed. In a large bowl, toss the pasta, pimientos and dressing together and adjust the seasoning to taste. Press the pasta into a large ring mould, allow to cool, then chill in the refrigerator for at least 1 hour.

Cut the chicken breasts into thin strips and stir-fry in the olive oil for 4-5 minutes or until the juices run clear but the chicken is still moist and soft.

Mix the coriander pesto with the chicken. Carefully turn out the pasta ring onto a serving platter and fill the centre with the pesto chicken. Garnish with coriander sprigs and serve.

Carrot-Ginger Mousse with Coriander Sauce

Ginger is traditionally regarded in Chinese medicine as a detoxificant – it is often used with potentially dangerous herbs to modify their action – and it also helps stimulate the digestion to cleanse the system. It is combined here with coriander (see page 120) and carrots which are an excellent tonic and cleansing food, traditionally used as a blood purifier in skin disorders.

Carrots are very stimulating for the digestion – the French herbalist, Jean Valnet describes them as *la grande amie de l'intestin*.

Serves 4

For the mousses:
1kg/2¼lb carrots
15g/½oz butter
200ml/7fl oz vegetable or chicken stock
25g/1oz fresh root ginger, peeled and grated
2 cloves garlic, crushed
2 eggs
½ teaspoon salt
½ teaspoon freshly ground black pepper

For the sauce:
1 bunch of fresh coriander, washed, dried and finely chopped
1 clove garlic, crushed
1–2 tablespoons lime juice
3 tablespoons olive oil
½ teaspoon salt
½ teaspoon freshly ground black pepper

Preheat the oven to 170°C/325°F/gas mark 3. First make the mousses. Peel the carrots and cut a few of them lengthwise into thin strips. Cook the strips in the melted butter and 55ml/2fl oz water until they become soft. Line the sides of 4 buttered ovenproof ramekin dishes with the carrot strips and set aside.

Slice the remaining carrots and boil them in the stock together with the ginger and garlic for 10-15 minutes, until tender. Drain well in a colander.

Blend the cooked vegetables and eggs in a blender or food processor until well mixed, then season to taste with salt and pepper. Divide the mousse equally between the ramekin dishes and bake in the oven for about 20 minutes, until the mousses are firm at the edges.

Meanwhile make the sauce by combining the coriander, garlic, lime juice and olive oil in a bowl. Whisk together until well mixed, then season to taste with salt and pepper.

When the mousses are cooked, turn them out on to serving plates, spoon a little of the sauce over each one and serve on their own as a starter or with a green salad for a light lunch.

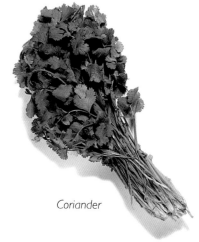

Coriander

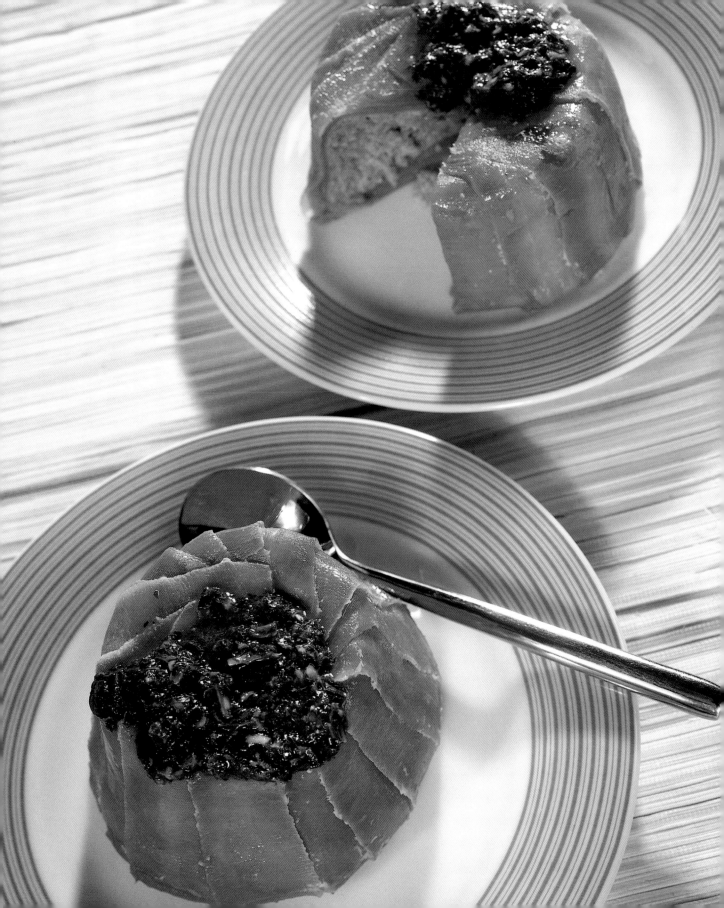

Bak Choy in Basil Oil Dressing

Just as cabbage is regarded in Western tradition as a cleansing and energising remedy for the digestive system (see Sauerkraut, page 136), so the various Chinese greens and cabbages are used in much the same way. Bak choy is a stimulating digestive remedy which is neutral, sweet and helpful for the large intestine and stomach.

In this dish, it is combined with basil oil which is also cleansing for the lower bowel, and a dash of chilli – a potent anti-microbial.

Serves 4

450g/1lb miniature bak choy

1 tablespoon basil oil (see Basics, page 188)

Dash of chilli sauce

Dash of maple syrup

½ teaspoon whole pink peppercorns (see page 96)

Salt

Steam the bak choy in a bamboo steamer for 6-7 minutes, until tender.

Mix together the basil oil, chilli sauce, maple syrup, peppercorns and salt to taste.

When the bak choy is ready, toss it in the dressing.

Serve with Pasta Ring with Coriander Pesto Chicken (see page 121) or Spiced Winter Lamb (see page 117).

The secret of true health lies in a strong immune system that will fight infection, orchestrate the body's own healing powers and even determine the rate at which we age. *Fu Zheng* therapy – which means to strengthen (*Fu*) the constitution (*Zheng*) – is the traditional Chinese equivalent of stimulating the immune system. *Fu Zheng* treatment can help to increase resistance to disease, prevent tissue damage, destroy abnormal cells and regulate body functions. Allergies, lethargy, repeated infection and slow wound healing are all signs of lowered immunity.

Just as poor nutrition weakens immunity, so the right foods can boost the body's natural defences. Strengthening herbs are also important – they are used to tonify *Qi*, *Jing* and Blood and to correct any deficiencies in these vital substances. Typical *Fu Zheng* herbs include *Huang Qi, Dang Shen, Ling Zhi* and *Ren Shen* (ginseng), as well as many which in the West we would regard as familiar foods – such as shiitake mushrooms and seaweeds. Some of these traditional remedies are specific to particular organs, helping to correct any weaknesses which may lead to ill health, while others are more general in their use.

Today, these herbs are also of value in combating the side-effects of potentially damaging Western medical techniques, such as chemotherapy and radiation which can weaken the immune system. Eat them regularly in these delicious soups and stews to strengthen the immune system and maintain health.

Building the Immune System

Ginseng and *Huang Qi* Mushroom Soup

This soup is a powerful *Qi* tonic to stimulate energy levels. It contains wood ear fungus (*Hei Mu Erh*), which is rich in amino acids (needed to build protein), phosphorus, iron, calcium and sugars. It was traditionally used, boiled in milk or beer, as a remedy for throat inflammations and is also an effective immune tonic. It also helps replenish *Jing* (essence).

The shiitake mushrooms (*Xiang Gu, Lentinus edodes*) have a proven anti-viral action and are an important and effective immune stimulant. Oyster mushrooms (*Pleurotus ostreatus,* known as *hiratake* in Japan) can be used instead of the shiitake. These are a traditional remedy used to ease tendon pains, but have more recently been shown to possess similar anti-tumour and immune-strengthening action to shiitake mushrooms.

Serves 6

25g/1oz *Hei Mu Erh*
1 onion, finely chopped
4 tablespoons olive oil
700g/1½lb fresh shiitake or
   oyster mushrooms, sliced
1.5 litres/2½ pints chicken or
   vegetable stock
15g/½oz *Ren Shen* (ginseng)
15g/½oz *Huang Qi*
Crème fraîche, to serve
2 tablespoons chopped fresh
   parsley, to garnish

Soak the *Hei Mu Erh* in water for 5-10 minutes to soften them, then rinse in clean water and set aside.

Sauté the onion in the oil for 2-3 minutes until it is soft and golden, then add the mushrooms and continue cooking for 3 minutes.

Add the stock, then the *Ren Shen*, *Huang Qi* and pre-soaked *Hei Mu Erh*. Bring to the boil, then reduce the heat, cover (leaving a small vent to allow the steam to escape) and simmer for 45 minutes.

Take the pan from the heat and remove the *Ren Shen* and *Huang Qi*. Allow to cool slightly, then purée the soup in a food processor or blender until smooth.

Return to the pan and warm through before serving garnished with a spoonful of crème fraîche and a little chopped parsley.

The *Ren Shen* may be chopped and served with the soup, rather like croutons, if desired, but the *Huang Qi* is too fibrous to eat and should be discarded.

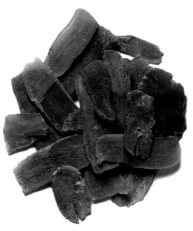

Ren Shen

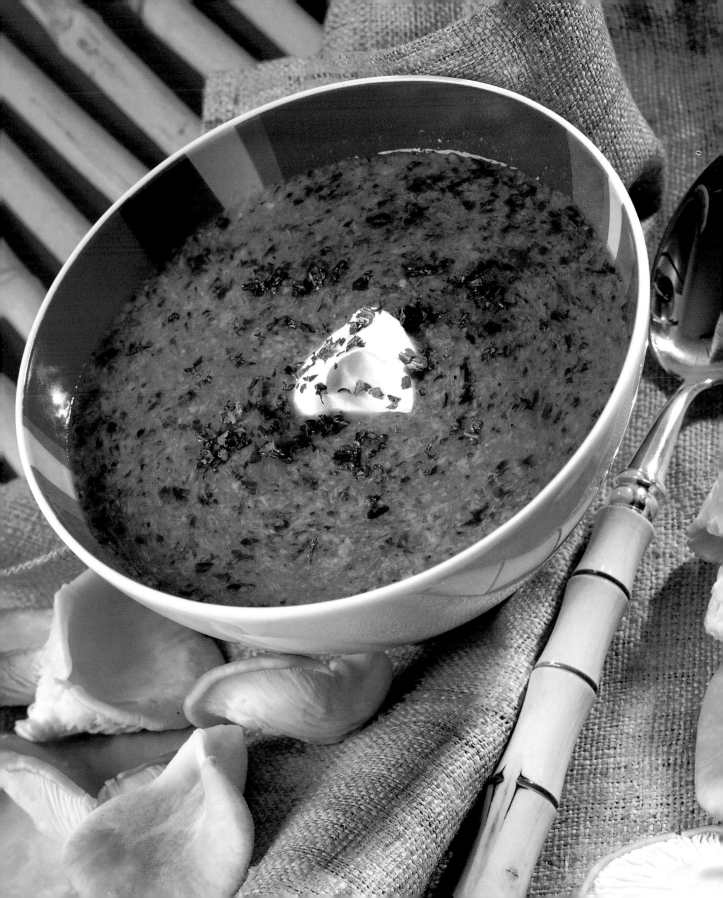

Shiitake Soup

Shiitake mushrooms (*Lentinus edodes*) – known in China as *Xiang Gu* or black mushrooms – contain several essential amino acids which are vital for building human protein. They also contain ergosterol, which is a provitamin and converts to vitamin D in sunlight, and a chemical called lentinan which is strongly anti-tumour.

Research has shown shiitake mushrooms, with their important essential amino acids, vitamins and minerals, to be one of our most readily available – and palatable – immune-stimulating foods. They are anti-viral, anti-tumour and protective for the liver. They are sweet and neutral and are traditionally said to tonify *Qi* and blood; they also benefit the stomach as well as soothing bronchial inflammations and normalising digestion in candida infections. As an anti-tumour remedy, they are especially effective in cases of stomach and cervical cancer.

Serves 4

55g/2oz dried shiitake mushrooms

225g/8oz fresh shiitake mushrooms

1 litre/1¾ pints chicken stock

Salt and freshly ground black pepper

Sprigs of fresh coriander, to garnish

Rinse the dried shiitake and soak them in hot water for 1 hour. Drain and be sure to keep both the shiitake and the strained liquid.

Remove the stems of both the dried and fresh shiitake and slice the caps. Put the dried shiitake and stock in a saucepan, bring to the boil, cover and simmer for 30 minutes. Remove the dried shiitake and save for use in another dish, as leaving them in this soup gives too strong a flavour.

Add the fresh mushrooms and the reserved liquid from soaking the dried mushrooms to the soup, bring to the boil and simmer gently for 10 minutes.

Season with salt and pepper and serve garnished with coriander sprigs.

Maize Pancakes with Ceps

Ceps *(Boletus edulis,)* have been a delicacy throughout Central Europe and China for centuries. In China, they are a key ingredient in traditional "tendon-easing pills" for back and joint pains and are classified as having a salty taste – suggesting a positive action on the kidneys.

Modern research has shown the mushrooms to be strongly anti-tumour, anti-inflammatory and strengthening for the immune system.

Although. like many wild mushrooms, fresh ceps are most readily available in the autumn, dried are now more easily obtainable from supermarkets. Soak the dried mushrooms in warm water for 10-20 minutes, then drain before use.

Serves 6

For the pancakes:
55g/2oz plain flour
115g/4oz maize flour
200ml/7fl oz milk
3 eggs, beaten
Pinch of salt
About 85g/3oz butter

For the stuffing:
3 onions, finely chopped
2 cloves garlic, crushed
450g/1lb fresh ceps, thinly sliced
1 dessertspoon olive oil
1 tablespoon chilli sauce
350g/12oz passata or 2 tablespoons tomato purée
1 teaspoon paprika
Pinch of salt
1 tablespoon finely chopped fresh flat-leaf parsley
1 tablespoon finely chopped fresh coriander
About 115g/4oz grated Parmesan cheese

To make the pancakes, sift the flours together and gradually beat in the milk. Beat in the eggs and salt to make a smooth batter, then leave to stand in the refrigerator for at least 30 minutes.

Preheat the oven to 200°C/400°F/gas mark 6. Make the stuffing by dry-frying the onion, garlic and ceps in a thick-based pan for about 6-8 minutes until the mixture is almost golden, shaking the pan during frying or stirring the mixture gently to prevent it sticking and burning.

Add the oil, chilli sauce, tomato purée, paprika, salt and herbs. Bring to the boil and simmer, uncovered, for about 5 minutes to reduce the liquid content. It should be a thick, spoonable mixture, not runny at all. Keep warm.

Remove the batter from the refrigerator and beat well. Melt a little of the butter in a frying pan and fry a ladleful of the batter to make a fairly thick pancake. Turn the pancake during cooking to brown both sides. The batter mixture is enough for 6 pancakes.

Place 2-3 tablespoons of the tomato and ceps mixture onto each pancake, sprinkle with 1 teaspoon Parmesan and roll them up. Place the pancake rolls seam side down in a greased baking dish. Sprinkle with the remaining Parmesan and bake in the oven for 10-15 minutes until the cheese is melted and golden. Serve with a green salad for lunch or supper.

Chanterelles and Chillies with Pasta

Like many mushrooms, chanterelles (*Cantharellus cibarius*) are rich in the eight kinds of amino acids that are essential for building human protein. They are also a good source of vitamin A so can be helpful for the eyes, reducing inflammation and abnormalities and improving night vision.

In traditional Chinese medicine, they are also believed to tonify the mucous membranes and combat dry skin. Studies also suggest that they can strengthen the immune system and combat respiratory infections.

Serves 4

200g/7oz dried chanterelles or 400g/14oz fresh chanterelles
1 tablespoon plus 1 teaspoon olive oil
2-3 cloves garlic, crushed
1-2 fresh chillies, deseeded and finely chopped
2 tablespoons sour cream
115g/4oz curd cheese
3 tablespoons *Huang Qi* brandy (see page 184)
Salt
500g/1lb 2oz fresh pasta such as tagliatelle or noodles
1 tablespoon chopped fresh parsley, to garnish

Soak the dried mushrooms in hot water for 10-15 minutes to restore the moisture content. Drain and reserve the liquid, which can be kept in a refrigerator for later use in stocks or stews. Slice the dried mushrooms and use as fresh. If using fresh mushrooms, rinse them in water, then drain and slice them.

Put the mushrooms in a dry saucepan over a low heat until the juices run, shaking the pan gently. Turn the heat up so that the liquid evaporates and the mushrooms are soft but reasonably dry.

Add 1 tablespoon oil to coat the mushrooms, then add the garlic, chillies, sour cream and curd cheese and let the mixture simmer over a low heat for 2-3 minutes. Add the *Huang Qi* brandy and season with a little salt to taste.

Meanwhile, cook the pasta in a large pan of salted, boiling water following the directions on the packet, until *al dente*. Add a teaspoon of olive oil to the water to prevent it boiling over and to enhance the flavour. Drain the pasta well.

Spoon the mushroom sauce over the pasta and garnish with parsley. Serve with a green salad for lunch or as a light supper dish.

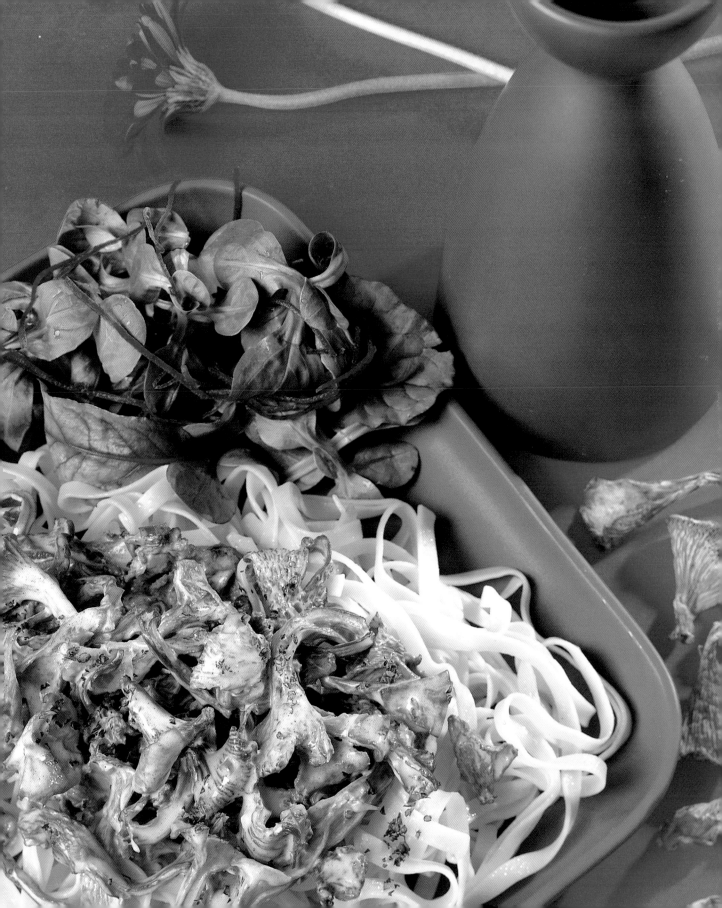

Spicy Liver Canapés

This warming liver dish makes a healthy winter cocktail party snack. It contains *Huang Qi,* stimulating for the immune system and *Qi,* coriander leaves which act as a detoxificant, with hot chilli and Sichuan peppercorns (*Hua Jiao, Zanthoxylum piperitum*). These are traditionally used for digestive problems especially spleen and stomach deficiency with abdominal pain, vomiting and diarrhoea. They also help to relieve pain and disperse cold – ideal winter food.

Makes about 50-60 canapés

1kg/2¼lb calves' liver, organically reared, left in one piece

15g/½oz *Huang Qi*

1 carrot, sliced

½ teaspoon Sichuan peppercorns

1 tablespoon olive oil

2 onions, sliced

5 fresh red chillies (fewer if you prefer a less hot taste), washed, deseeded and sliced into long thin strips

5 cloves garlic, crushed

Salt

3 tablespoons chopped fresh coriander

Rinse the liver in cold water until it runs clear. Put the *Huang Qi* into a large pan of water and bring to the boil. Immerse the whole slab of liver in the boiling water, add the carrot and boil for about 20-30 minutes. Add half the Sichuan peppercorns in the last 5 minutes of cooking.

Remove the pan from the heat and leave the liver to cool in the liquid. When it is cool enough to handle, remove it from the liquid and slice it into 5mm/¼in thick slices, then cut through the slices to make 2.5cm/1in squares. Discard the *Huang Qi,* but reserve the strained cooking liquid and use as stock in soups and stews.

Heat the oil in a wok or frying pan and sauté the onions for 3-4 minutes until they begin to colour, then add the chillies and garlic. Stir well, then add the liver pieces. Sauté gently for about 10 minutes – taking care not to damage your liver squares – until the liver is infused with the spice flavours.

Add salt to taste and grind a few more of the Sichuan peppercorns into the mixture if you like the taste, which is strongly aromatic. Stir in the coriander and serve with cocktail sticks as canapés.

Chicken Stir-Fry with Ceps

Chicken is classed as sweet and warm and helps to stimulate the spleen and stomach, while the ceps *(Boletus edulis)* are a good immune stimulant and have shown anti-tumour properties in trials. The shiitake, too, will also stimulate the immune system, while green vegetables help provide essential vitamins and minerals.

This dish is ideal to tonify the digestion and help combat seasonal winter chills.

Serves 4

25g/1oz dried ceps

1 large courgette

115-175g/4-6oz broccoli

115g/4oz fine French beans, trimmed

3-4 skinless, boneless chicken breasts (depending on size and appetites)

2 tablespoons groundnut oil

2 cloves garlic, crushed

2.5cm/1in piece fresh root ginger, peeled and finely chopped

55g/2oz fresh shiitake mushrooms, sliced

2 tablespoons Chinese cooking wine, rice wine or sherry

1 tablespoon soy sauce

150ml/¼ pint chicken stock

1 teaspoon cornflour, stirred into a paste with a little water

Cover the dried ceps with hot water and soak for 10-15 minutes. Slice the courgette lengthways, then cut into strips and finally into rectangular pieces about 5cm/2in long. Set aside.

Cut the broccoli into small florets and the stem into small chunks. Steam the beans and broccoli for 5-6 minutes or until tender. Drain, set aside and keep warm.

Cut the chicken into long strips about 1-2cm/½-¾in wide. Heat the oil in a wok and stir-fry the garlic and ginger for 1 minute, then add the chicken and stir-fry for 7-8 minutes.

Drain the ceps and add them with the shiitake mushrooms and courgettes to the chicken. Stir-fry for a further 4-5 minutes, then add the wine, rice wine or sherry and soy sauce and mix well.

Add the stock and cornflour mixture and stir-fry until the sauce thickens, mixing well so that the chicken and vegetables are well coated in the sauce. Add the cooked beans and broccoli and stir to coat them in the sauce.

Serve immediately with plain boiled brown rice or noodles.

Ginger-Marinated Chicken

Fresh ginger is warming in nature and it is used here with lime, garlic and honey which help to increase resistance and strengthen the immunity: an ideal combination to fight the first signs of a cold, helping to combat symptoms and stimulate circulation. Reduce the quantity of paprika and garlic if you prefer less strongly flavoured food.

Serves 4–5

4 tablespoons soy sauce

1 heaped tablespoon chopped fresh root ginger

3-5 cloves garlic, crushed

Finely grated zest and juice of 1-2 limes

3 tablespoons clear honey

1 free-range chicken, about 1.5kg/3½lb in weight

1-1½kg/2-3lb potatoes

½-1 teaspoon salt

½-1 tablespoon paprika

½ teaspoon freshly ground black pepper

Mix the soy sauce, ginger, garlic, lime zest and juice and honey together. Cut the chicken into 8-10 pieces and marinate them in the lime mixture in a covered container for 8-12 hours, or overnight in the refrigerator.

Preheat the oven to 220°C/425°F/gas mark 7. Peel the potatoes, cut them into thin rounds, place them in an ovenproof dish and sprinkle with the salt, paprika and pepper. Place the chicken pieces on top of the potatoes, then pour over the remaining marinade.

Cover and bake in the oven for about 1 hour or until the chicken is cooked, the juices run clear and the potatoes are tender.

Serve with Broccoli and Brussels Sprout Warmer (see page 42).

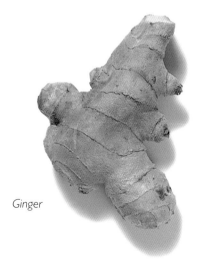

Ginger

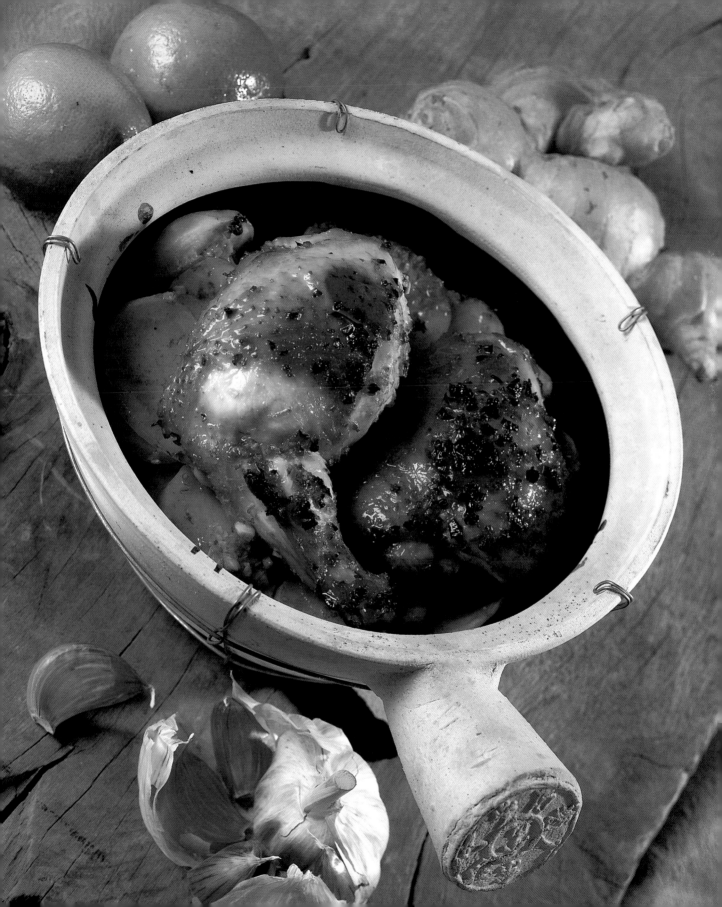

Stuffed Sauerkraut Leaves

Sauerkraut – fermented cabbage – is eaten throughout central and eastern Europe in winter. It dates from the days before refrigeration, when the only way to keep the cabbage crop through the winter was to ferment it in wooden casks.

Sauerkraut is rich in vitamin C, which helps combat infection, and contains a type of lactic acid which helps the digestion by clearing harmful bacteria and combating toxins, food stagnation and wind. Some researchers also maintain that, due to its lactic acid content, it is an effective preventative for cancer and degenerative diseases. It also stimulates and nourishes the liver and is well known in parts of Europe as an unsurpassed home remedy for hangovers.

In this dish, whole sauerkraut leaves are used. They can sometimes be found in Polish or Italian delicatessens; if not, use ordinary unfermented cabbage leaves (as described in the recipe) and add shredded sauerkraut, which is readily available in supermarkets. If you want to ferment your own whole cabbage, follow the instructions at the end of the recipe.

Serves 4

For the stuffed sauerkraut leaves:

8 whole sauerkraut leaves, or 8 whole fresh cabbage leaves (plus a pinch of salt, 2 teaspoons wine vinegar and 6 black peppercorns)

1 tablespoon olive oil

2 onions, thinly sliced

3 cloves garlic, crushed

450g/1lb minced meat (pork, beef or a mixture of the two)

125g/4½oz long-grain rice, washed

2 teaspoons paprika

2 tablespoons chopped fresh parsley

Salt and freshly ground black pepper

Whole sauerkraut leaves simply need to have the stalks trimmed. If using fresh cabbage, carefully remove 8 leaves from the stem. Some cabbage varieties have rather thick veins in the back, if so trim them off so that the leaf bends more easily.

Bring a large pan of water to the boil and add a pinch of salt, two teaspoons wine vinegar and 6 black peppercorns. Put the leaves into the water, two at a time, and cook for a few minutes. Watch carefully and remove the leaves as soon as they begin to wilt. Set aside to drain on absorbent kitchen paper.

To make the stuffing, heat the oil in a frying pan and sauté the onions and garlic for 2-3 minutes until softened. Add the minced meat and cook for 5-6 minutes until it is lightly browned all over. Add the rice, paprika and parsley and mix well. Cook for 2-3 minutes, then remove from the heat and set aside to cool. Season to taste with salt and pepper.

When the stuffing has cooled to a manageable temperature, place some of the mixture on the centre of each sauerkraut leaf and fold up into small parcels. Secure with kitchen string or cocktail sticks if necessary.

Put a layer of shredded sauerkraut in the bottom of a saucepan, place the cabbage parcels on top and finish with the smoked pork or bacon.

310g/11oz shredded sauerkraut

310g/11oz smoked rib of pork or smoked bacon, chopped

For the sauce:
1 tablespoon olive oil
3 teaspoons plain flour
Salt and a few black peppercorns
20g/¾oz tomato purée
1 small chilli, finely chopped
150ml/¼ pint beef stock
115g/4oz crème fraîche

Carefully add enough water to reach above the middle of the layers. If necessary, weigh the parcels down with a small plate.

Bring to the boil, then simmer on a gentle heat for 2 hours making sure that the mixture does not go dry. Top the water level up from time to time to keep it just below the top layer of cabbage parcels, about three-quarters of the way up the ingredients.

Meanwhile, make the sauce by heating the oil in a small saucepan, adding the flour and cooking until lightly browned, stirring. Add salt to taste, a few peppercorns, tomato purée and chilli, then add enough beef stock to make a sauce with the consistency of single cream.

Add the sauce to the pan containing the parcels, bring to the boil and simmer for a further 15-20 minutes. Serve topped with crème fraîche.

Preserving Whole Cabbage Heads

This is a traditional late-October task in many parts of Europe. Instead of the original wooden casks, use food-grade plastic tubs fitted with a tap for draining the water. Once filled with cabbage, the tubs will need to be stored in a cold cellar – preferably one where the smell of fermenting cabbage will not prove too invasive.

Clean the cabbages, removing the stems and slightly hollowing the cut ends. Layer in the tub with the scooped-out bases uppermost. Pour salt into the base opening of each cabbage head and cover with a linen cloth. Weigh down the cabbages in the tub with a plate so that they will not rise up out of the water and then pour in enough fresh water to cover the cabbages completely.

During the first week, drain off the water twice using the tap in the fermenting tub. Wash the linen cloth and weights separately and replace. Refill the tub with fresh water and top up if necessary. Cabbage brine is an esteemed traditional tonic, rich in vitamin C and taken to combat fatigue and infection.

Depending on the temperature of the cellar, it usually takes several weeks before fermentation is completed. The cabbage leaves should be firm but pliable. The large outer leaves can be used in the above recipe, while the cabbage hearts can be shredded and used in salads or as you would use chopped sauerkraut. Store in brine in jars. Once out of the brine it will keep in a closed container in the refrigerator for a day or two.

Rolled Sole with Oyster Mushrooms

Oyster mushrooms (*Pleurotus ostreatus,* known as *hiratake* in Japan) are a good source of essential amino acids. They are defined as sweet and mild in Chinese medicine and were traditionally used to strengthen veins, relax the tendons and ease aching limbs. More recent studies have highlighted their anti-cancer properties and they will also help to reduce cholesterol levels in blood, as well as helping to strengthen and improve the immune system.

Serves 4

225g/8oz oyster mushrooms
25g/1oz butter
Salt and freshly ground black pepper
1 tablespoon chopped fresh tarragon
8 fillets of lemon sole, washed, dried and skinned
1 teaspoon cornflour
275ml/½ pint fish stock
120ml/4fl oz dry white wine

Preheat the oven to 190°C/375°F/gas mark 5. Oyster mushrooms should not be washed, just wiped with a clean kitchen towel. Separate the mushroom cups, trim off the stems and slice the mushrooms.

Melt the butter in a frying pan and sauté the mushrooms over a medium heat for about 5 minutes, then season with salt and pepper and add half the tarragon. Remove the pan from the heat.

Sprinkle salt and pepper over each fish fillet and lay them flesh side down on a board. Spread a layer of sautéed mushrooms over each fillet, roll them up and secure with fine kitchen thread or wooden cocktail sticks. Place the rolled fillets in a buttered ovenproof dish.

Mix the cornflour and a little fish stock into a paste, then add the rest of the stock and wine and pour over the fish rolls. Cover the dish tightly with foil and bake in the oven for 20-30 minutes, depending on the size of the fillets. The fish should be opaque when cooked.

Garnish with the remaining tarragon. Serve with plain boiled rice and mangetout or green beans.

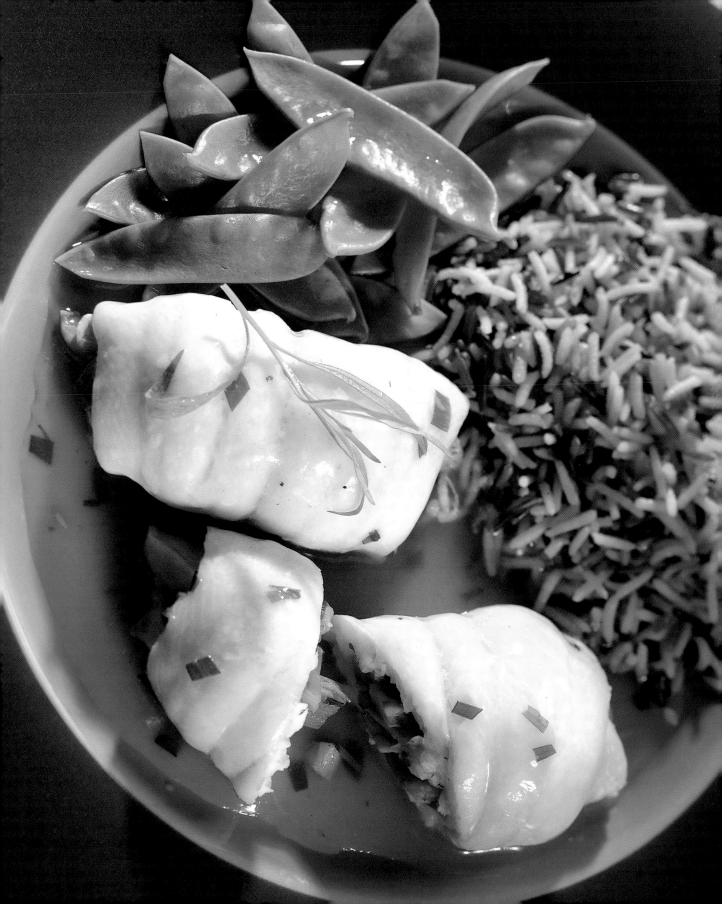

The mythical Chinese Yellow Emperor *(Huang Di),* who reputedly lived around 2500BC, maintained that men's lives were counted in groups of eight years and women's in seven: by the time each reached 56 or 49 respectively, vital essence *(Jing)* and reproductive energies had been seriously eroded and old age began.

The Western view of the "third age" is rather more optimistic than the Yellow Emperor's, but it can still be helped by suitable tonics to strengthen *Jing* and kidney *Qi* which the Chinese associate with the symptoms of ageing. Kidney energy is also associated with the reproductive system and sexuality so many of these tonics are also classified as aphrodisiac.

Most of the recipes in this section will act as energising tonics for those in their "middle" and "third" ages – but some will also have a distinct effect on libido…

Rejuvenating Dishes for All Ages

Longevity Noodles

Long noodles in Chinese culture represent long life and are a speciality served at celebration feasts. Great care should be taken not to cut the noodles, which would be very unlucky.

The *Gou Qi Zi* (lycii berries) help to replenish liver and kidney *yin,* so are ideal at combating many of the symptoms of ageing, such as failing eyesight, lower back pain and tiredness. Black sesame seeds are especially invigorating for liver and kidney, and so are an ideal nourishing food for the elderly.

Serves 4

115g/4oz mung bean sprouts
225g/8oz dried egg noodles
Salt
275ml/½ pint chicken or
 vegetable stock
1 teaspoon shoyu soy sauce
½ teaspoon sesame seed oil
1 tablespoon walnut oil
1cm/½in piece fresh root
 ginger, peeled and sliced
115g/4oz mangetout
55g/2oz *Gou Qi Zi*, washed
3 large fresh water
 chestnuts, peeled and
 sliced (use canned if fresh
 are not available)
1 tablespoon black sesame
 seeds

Blanch the mung bean sprouts in a pan of boiling water for 10 seconds, then drain and refresh with cold water. Drain again and set aside. Cook the egg noodles in salted water for 1 minute, then drain and refresh with cold water. Lift gently with a fork to separate and dry. Keep warm.

Mix together the stock, shoyu and sesame oil to make a sauce. Set aside.

Put the walnut oil and the ginger in a hot wok, then add the mangetout and *Gou Qi Zi* and stir-fry for 1 minute. Add the water chestnuts and finally the bean sprouts. Stir-fry for 1 minute. Pour in the sauce, bring to the boil and stir-fry for 2 minutes.

Meanwhile, heat the black sesame seeds in a clean, dry pan until warm. Pour the vegetable sauce over the noodles and sprinkle with the warm sesame seeds. Serve immediately.

Pumpkin Seeds Tossed in Soy Sauce

450g/1lb pumpkin seeds
5-6 tablespoons shoyu soy
 sauce

Try these as an alternative garnish to sesame seeds. Pumpkin seeds are rich in zinc and so help to prevent prostate cancer.

Preheat the oven to 220°C/425°F/gas mark 7. In a bowl, toss together the pumpkin seeds and enough soy sauce to coat them all over. Place in a roasting pan and cook in the oven for about 10 minutes, until the seeds are slightly browned and a little sticky. Set aside to cool. Store the pumpkin seeds in a clean storage jar and eat one large handful a day or use to sprinkle on salads and noodles.

Tonic Duck Soup

Dong Chong Xia Cao (caterpillar fungus) is one of the most important Chinese *Qi* tonics which helps to restore lung and kidney *Qi* and *Jing*. It was once very rare and reserved exclusively for the Chinese Emperors and their families, who would eat duck stuffed with fungus and then roasted. Today, the fungus is often grown on a grain base (rather than caterpillars) and so its amazing restorative powers can be enjoyed by all.

Cooking it with duck or chicken is believed to increase its potency and also makes an especially restorative soup for chronic respiratory problems, such as bronchitis. It also helps to combat kidney energy weakness, which in Chinese theory may be associated with back pains, night sweats or sexual problems. The fungus is one of the best tonics for strengthening *Jing* (essence), which is often depleted in the elderly.

Serves 4-6

1 duck, about 1.3kg/3lb in weight, skinned
25g/1oz *Dong Chong Xia Cao*
1 tablespoon soy sauce
2 litres/3½ pints water or vegetable or chicken stock
115g/4oz spinach or rocket, chopped and lightly steamed for 2-3 minutes
Salt and freshly ground black pepper

Put the duck into a saucepan with the *Dong Chong Xia Cao* and sprinkle with soy sauce. Add the water or stock and bring to the boil, then cover and simmer for 3 hours, or until the meat falls from the carcass.

Remove the pan from the heat and remove and discard the bones and carcass. Break the duck meat into smaller pieces.

Add the spinach or rocket leaves, stir well and season to taste with salt and pepper. Serve with crusty French bread.

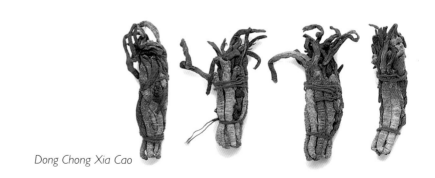

Dong Chong Xia Cao

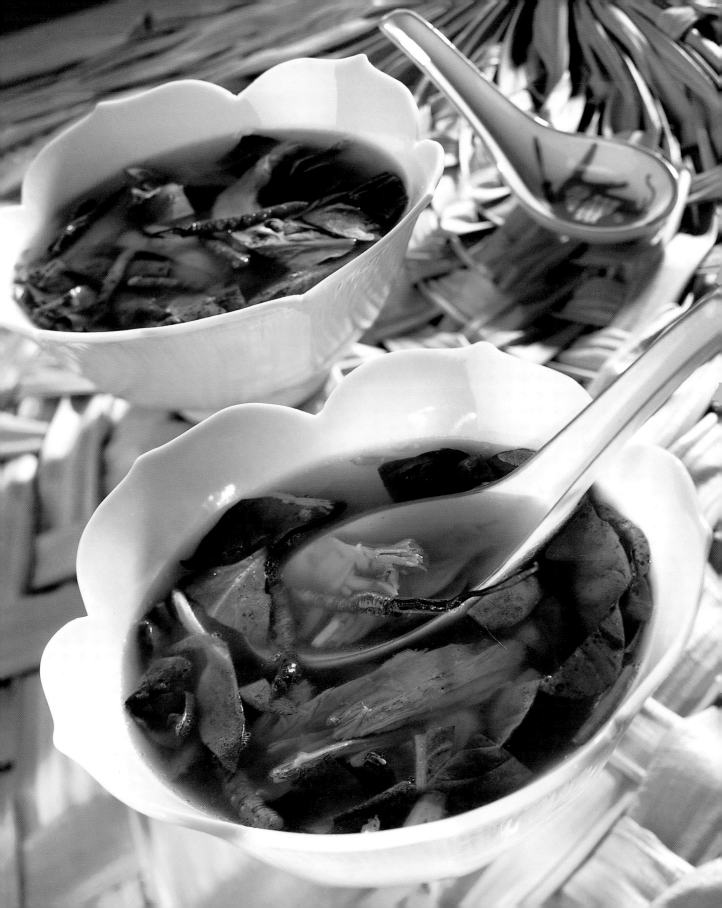

Duck Stuffed with Ginseng and Rice

This recipe invigorates the *Qi* and replenishes the spleen. It is good for weakness and tiredness.

Duck tonifies *Qi*, blood and *yin* and nourishes and lubricates the body. In China, ducks are symbols of happiness and when they are found in pairs they indicate conjugal fidelity.

Lian Zi (lotus seeds) are neutral with a sweet flavour. They nourish the heart, tonify the kidney and spleen, and are also astringent for the intestines. The seeds can be bought dried or pre-cooked. To prepare the dried seeds, soak them in water for 10 minutes, drain, then boil in fresh water for 10 minutes. Pre-cooked seeds need no preparation.

Pine nuts are sweet and warm and they moisturise the lungs, lubricate the intestinal tract and encourage production of body fluids (*Jin-Ye*). Ginseng (*Ren Shen* – see page 64) is one of the most important of the Chinese energy tonics.

Serves 2

- **115g/4oz wild rice**
- **25g/1oz Lian Zi (prepared as above)**
- **10g/⅓oz ginseng (or substitute Dang Shen, which is less expensive)**
- **55g/2oz pine nuts**
- **2 Spanish onions, chopped**
- **2 teaspoons sesame seed oil, plus extra to brown the duck**
- **1 clove garlic, peeled**
- **1 slice root ginger, peeled**
- **3 tablespoons hoisin sauce**
- **3 teaspoons soy sauce**
- **1 tablespoon sherry or rice wine**
- **1 tablespoon clear honey**
- **Salt and black pepper**
- **½ teaspoon Chinese five-spice powder (Wu Xiang Fen)**
- **1 boned duck, skin left on, about 1.3kg/3lb (ask the butcher to bone it for you)**

Cover the wild rice with 2.5cm/1in water in a saucepan, add the *Lian Zi* and ginseng, bring to the boil and cook for about 20 minutes until the grains are just bursting. Add the pine nuts, remove the pan from the heat, drain if necessary and set aside.

Sauté the onion gently in 2 teaspoons sesame oil until golden. Mince the garlic and ginger together and add to the onions with the hoisin sauce, 2 teaspoons soy sauce, the sherry or rice wine, honey, salt and pepper and five-spice powder, mixing well. Stir this into the rice mixture and mix well.

Lay out the boned duck skin side down on a board. Spread the rice filling evenly over the open duck. Using cooking thread or cocktail sticks lace or secure the edges of the duck together.

Rub the duck with the remaining soy sauce and fry in a large pan in a little sesame oil, turning the duck until it is browned all over.

Cover the duck with boiling water, place a lid on the pan, bring to the boil, then simmer slowly for about 4 hours. The duck will become puffed and tender. Serve on a bed of steamed purple-sprouting broccoli.

Lamb's Kidneys with Basil and Tomato

Lamb's kidneys in traditional Chinese medicine are – perhaps not surprisingly – seen as restorative and strengthening food for our own kidneys. They are warming with a sweet taste to tonify *yang*, *Qi* and blood. They also benefit *Jing* (essence, see page 12) so are especially suitable as we head for the third age and *Jing* levels are depleted. Kidneys also move stagnant blood (see page 84) and *Qi* and are often eaten for weaknesses associated with the kidney – such as low back pain, hearing problems, impotence, excessive urination and weak legs.

In this dish, the kidneys are combined with tomatoes – which modern research has shown to act as a preventative for certain sorts of cancer, especially prostate disorders, as well as basil, a stimulating and energising herb, coriander and thyme. This meal is ideal as a generally energising dish but can be especially helpful for menopausal problems and in old age.

Serves 4

8-12 lamb's kidneys (depending on size and appetites)
1-2 tablespoons seasoned plain flour
2 tablespoons olive oil
3 cloves garlic, crushed
450g/1lb passata, or use 400g/14oz can chopped Italian tomatoes, preferably organic
1 teaspoon ground coriander
2 teaspoons chopped fresh thyme
Pinch of granulated sugar
Salt and freshly ground black pepper
8 large fresh basil leaves
175g/6oz fresh shiitake mushrooms, quartered
120ml/4fl oz sherry

Remove and discard the outer membrane from the kidneys, cut them into quarters and remove the central core – it is easiest to do this with kitchen scissors. Toss the kidneys in the flour until they are well coated.

Heat ½ tablespoon oil in a small saucepan and sauté the garlic for 2-3 minutes so that it is softened but not browned. Add the passata or chopped tomatoes, coriander, thyme, sugar and seasoning. If using chopped tomatoes, stir well to crush them further. Bring to the boil and then reduce to a steady simmer. Partially cover the mixture with a lid as the tomato sauce tends to spit. Cook for 15-20 minutes until you have a thick spoonable sauce which should not be watery at all. When the sauce is cooked, stir the shredded basil into the mixture. Keep warm.

Meanwhile, heat 1 tablespoon oil in a separate frying pan or wok and sauté the mushrooms for 4-5 minutes. Remove from the pan to a warmed serving dish, set aside and keep warm.

Add the remaining oil to the pan if necessary and stir-fry the kidney quarters for 3-4 minutes, until they are well browned but not over-cooked or they will become tough. Pour the sherry into the pan and allow it to bubble vigorously for 1-2 minutes to evaporate the alcohol. Return the mushrooms to the pan, add the tomato sauce and mix well. Add more salt and pepper if required and return the mixture to the warmed serving dish. Serve with plain boiled rice and spinach.

Longevity Pork Stew

This combination of herbs and pork will tonify the *Qi*, nourish kidney *yin* and tonify blood, so it is an ideal dish for older people, helping to restore basic energy and *Jing* (essence – see page 12). Walnut oil is a good source of essential fatty acids, which boost the metabolism and help combat ageing.

Bai He (lily bulb) is especially strengthening for lung yin, *Shan Yao* (Chinese yam) helps to invigorate spleen, stomach, lung and kidney as well as helping *Jing* (essence) while *Huang Qi* helps *Wei Qi* (defence energy), spleen and lung so this dish is also ideal in convalescence.

The Chinese prefer pork above other meats, not only because it is extremely tasty but also because pigs are lazy and spend their days in comfort, sleeping and eating. This stew is best eaten on the second day.

Serves 4-6

1kg/2lb stewing pork, cut into 2.5cm/1in cubes
4 tablespoons rice wine
2 tablespoons chopped fresh chives
2 tablespoons chopped fresh coriander
2 tablespoons walnut oil
2 tablespoons brown sugar
15g/½oz *Bai He* (lily bulb)
15g/½oz *Shan Yao* (Chinese yam)
15g/½oz *Gou Qi Zi* (lycii berries)
2 pieces *Huang Qi*
55g/2oz fresh shiitake mushrooms, quartered
½ carrot, sliced
2 leeks, washed and sliced
1 large potato, sliced
Salt and freshly ground black pepper
2 tablespoons chopped fresh coriander and chives, to garnish

Marinate the pork in the rice wine, chives and coriander, ideally overnight but for at least 4 hours.

Heat the oil in a large saucepan, then add the sugar. Continue heating until the sugar softens, but before it starts to bubble and burn, add the pork pieces. Brown the pork all over to seal the meat. Add the marinade, the Chinese herbs, shiitake mushrooms, carrot, leeks and potato. Sauté gently for 2-3 minutes, then add 150ml/¼ pint water.

Cover, bring to the boil and simmer over a low heat for about 2 hours or until the meat is tender. Check regularly that there is enough liquid in the pan and add a little more water if required.

When cooked, the dish will improve by being left in a cool place for 24 hours before use and then reheated thoroughly. Season to taste before serving.

Remove and discard the pieces of *Huang Qi* and serve the stew on a bed of boiled rice or noodles, garnished with coriander and chives.

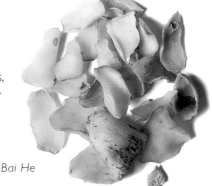

Bai He

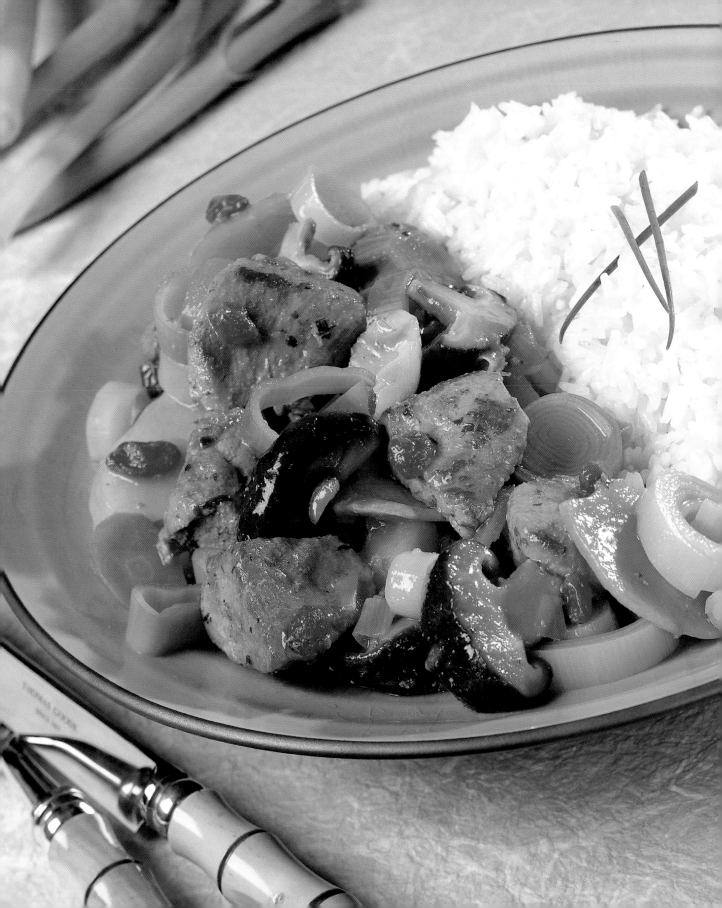

Preserving Youth Jelly

Amachazuru (Gynostemma pentaphyllum), also known in Japan as gospel herb, is an anti-ageing immune stimulant which has been shown to increase cell activity and so act as a preventative for cancer. It has also been used in recent years for the prevention and treatment of cardiovascular diseases, diabetes, asthma and bronchitis. *Amachazuru* is an effective tonic to combat fatigue as well as a relaxant for the whole system. In the West, it is sold mainly in tea bags.

Agar-agar *(Gellidium amausii, Dong Fen)* is refined from seaweed and gives a clear firm jelly.

Serves 4

5 *amachazuru* tea bags
2 teaspoons agar-agar
   powder
85g/3oz granulated sugar
A few drops of rose or
   jasmine essence
Crème fraîche, to serve
   (optional)

Pour about 500ml/1 pint hot water onto the *amachazuru* tea bags to make a strong infusion. Leave to steep for 20 minutes.

Pour the strained tea into a saucepan and sprinkle the agar-agar powder over the surface. Bring slowly to the boil and stir until the agar-agar has dissolved. Add the sugar and stir until dissolved.

Remove the pan from the heat and stir in the flower essence, then pour the mixture into individual jelly moulds or bowls. Set aside to cool, then leave to set for a few hours in the refrigerator.

Serve with crème fraîche, if you like.

Double Boiled Chicken with *Gou Qi Zi* and *Dong Chong Xia Cao*

This nourishing chicken dish combines *Gou Qi Zi* (lycii berries) and *Dong Chong Xia Cao* (caterpillar fungus), which are both ideal herbs to restore failing energies in the third age. The chicken and red dates *(Hong Zao)* are warming, while the dates are also a traditional remedy for building strength and easing the rheumatic aches and pains of old age.

The chicken is steamed in its own juices for 4 hours.

Serves 4

1 free-range chicken, weighing about 1.3kg/3lb, gizzard and neck reserved
55g/2oz salt
25g/1oz *Dong Chong Xia Cao*
8 Chinese red dates (*Hong Zao*)
25g/1oz *Gou Qi Zi*
1 teaspoon shoyu soy sauce

Rub the chicken all over with the salt, then rinse under cold water and pat dry. Put the chicken in a large heat-proof bowl and add the gizzard, neck, *Dong Chong Xia Cao*, red dates and *Gou Qi Zi*. Cover with a lid or heatproof plate.

Place the bowl in a steamer, or use a cake rack placed inside a large saucepan. Add 10cm/4in boiling water to the saucepan and cover. Boil for 4 hours or until the chicken is extremely tender, making sure there is always enough boiling water in the pan and topping up as necessary.

Lift the chicken from the bowl and remove and discard the skin. Separate the chicken meat from the bones and discard the bones, gizzard and neck.

Divide the chicken between 4 individual soup bowls. Pour over the cooking juices, dates and *Gou Qi Zi* and serve sprinkled with a little shoyu.

Serve with crusty French bread or croutons. You can eat the *Dong Chong Xia Cao* or not, as preferred.

Pork Chops with *Shi Hu*

Shi Hu (orchid stem) was a favourite with the ancient Taoists who used it in a daily tea or – when in season – as a fresh vegetable. The herb is believed to replenish *Jing* (vital essence, see page 12) and strengthen kidney *yin,* so helping to combat the effects of ageing. It is also said to increase sexual vigour and combat fatigue associated with excessive sexual activity.

As a potent kidney tonic, *Shi Hu* also relieves lower back and knee pains, as well as helping to restore body fluids (*Jin-Ye*) and acts as a restorative in debility and convalescence. *Shi Hu* is also said to supply "healing energy" so is an ideal restorative tonic for people involved in the healing arts.

In this recipe, it is used with pork (see page 146) which is also a good *Qi* and blood tonic which tonifies *yin.*

Kaffir lime leaves can be found in many supermarkets. They are glossy and thick, rather like bay leaves, with an aromatic citrus scent and are used whole and fresh, if possible. Like bay leaves they are to supply flavour – not to eat.

Serves 4

20g/¾oz *Shi Hu*
4 medium pork chops
Salt and black pepper
1 dessertspoon olive oil
2 cloves garlic, crushed
3 teaspoons cornflour
2 teaspoons paprika
1 teaspoon vegetable
** bouillon or 1 stock cube**
6 kaffir lime leaves

Preheat the oven to 190°C/375°F/gas mark 5. Chop any large pieces of dried *Shi Hu* and cover the stems with about 500ml/1 pint water. Bring to the boil, cover the pan and simmer for 10-15 minutes. Remove the pan from the heat and leave to cool.

Rub the chops all over with salt and pepper. Fry them in a lightly oiled frying pan for about 10 minutes, turning once, until both sides are slightly browned. Remove the chops from the pan and transfer to a casserole dish.

Add the garlic to the pan juices and sauté for a few seconds, mixing well. Sprinkle the cornflour and paprika into the pan and continue stirring over a low heat.

Strain the liquid in which the *Shi Hu* were boiled and add this to the frying pan. Discard the *Shi Hu.* Add the vegetable bouillon or stock cube and lime leaves to the pan and bring to the boil, stirring. Adjust the seasoning to taste.

Pour the sauce over the chops, cover and cook in the oven for about 20 minutes, or until the chops are cooked and tender. Serve with Love-in-a-Mist Potatoes (see page 152) or Mashed Potatoes with Sesame Seeds (see page 104). Remove the lime leaves before serving.

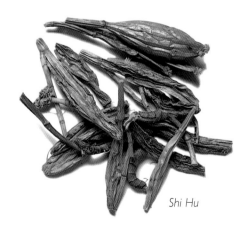

Shi Hu

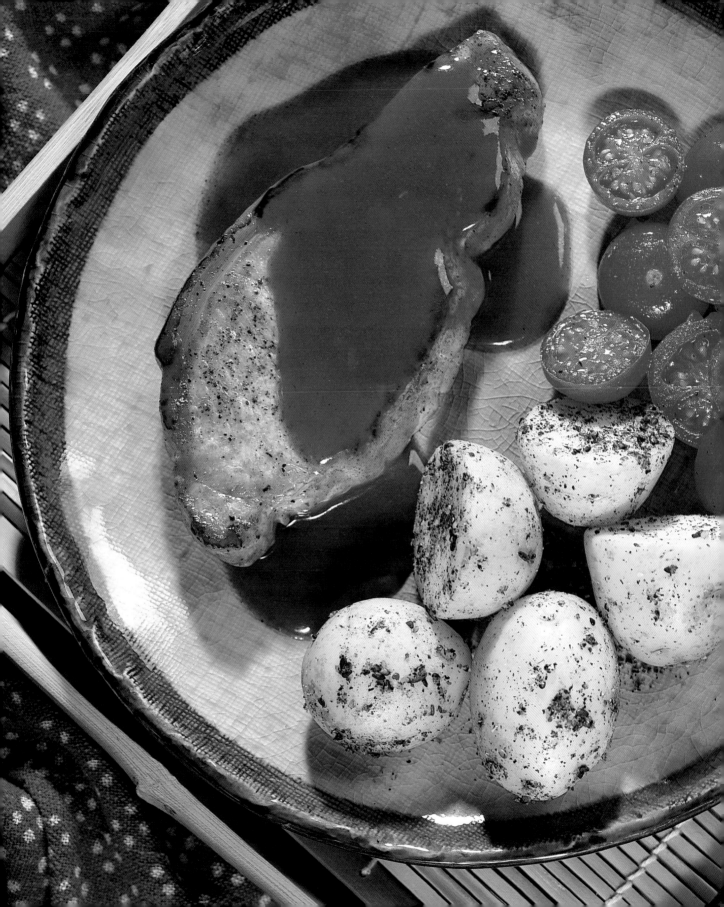

Prawn and Walnut Stir-Fry

Walnuts are a warming, *yang* tonic for the kidneys, which in Chinese medicine are closely associated with reproduction and sexuality. They are combined here with prawns or shrimps (also stimulating and *yang*) and bak choy (*Xiao Baicai*) which is classified as sweet, neutral and *yang*. The result is a stimulating mixture to invigorate the reproductive organs.

Serves 4

450g/1lb bak choy

150ml/¼ pint chicken stock

1 tablespoon arrowroot or kuzu

2 teaspoons shoyu soy sauce

1 teaspoon sesame seed oil

1 thumb-size piece fresh root ginger, peeled

2 cloves garlic

2 shallots

1 spring onion

2 tablespoons walnut oil

225g/8oz prawns or shrimps, shells and veins removed

55g/2oz shelled walnuts

1 tablespoon fresh coriander leaves

Blanch the bak choy in a large saucepan of boiling water for 20 seconds, then drain and rinse under cold water. Set aside. Mix together the stock, arrowroot or kuzu, half the shoyu and half the sesame oil. Set aside.

Put the ginger, garlic, shallots and spring onion in a food processor and process until finely chopped.

Stir-fry the ginger and garlic mixture in a hot wok with the remaining sesame oil for about 2 minutes or until it smells strong and nutty and turns a golden brown, then add the remaining shoyu. Remove from the wok and put to one side.

Heat the walnut oil in the wok, add the prawns or shrimps and bak choy and stir-fry for 2 minutes, then add the roughly chopped walnuts, the stock mixture and the ginger mixture and stir-fry until hot.

Serve garnished with coriander as a starter or with boiled noodles or rice for a more substantial course.

Love-in-a-Mist Potatoes

Serves 4

450g/1lb new potatoes in their skins

3 tablespoons sesame seeds

1 tablespoon flaked almonds

½ teaspoon sea salt

1 teaspoon black cumin seeds (see page 73)

Cook the potatoes in a pan of boiling water for 15-20 minutes until tender. Drain.

In a thick-based pan, dry-fry the sesame seeds and almonds with the sea salt, taking care not to burn them. As soon as they turn golden, add the black cumin (love-in-a-mist), stir and remove from the heat. Chop the toasted seeds and nuts in a blender or food processor until the almonds are well crushed. Toss the hot potatoes in the seed mixture and serve.

Pigeon Love Stew

Pigeon, known in China as *Pak Cap* or *baak gup,* is used to tonify the blood, remove excess dampness and nurture *Qi* and blood after childbirth. However, by far the most common use for pigeon meat is to combat male impotence by strengthening blood and *Qi*. It is also regarded as an excellent kidney tonic, so is a popular choice for regular eating.

Symbolically, doves and pigeons represent impartiality, peace, longevity, conjugal faithfulness and filial duty – eating them is also believed to impart some of these properties. The meat is lean, fragrant, nutritious and tender.

In this recipe, *Dang Gui* (Chinese angelica) and *Dang Shen* are added to enhance the *Qi* and blood tonifying action.

Serves 4

4 whole oven-ready pigeons, each about 225g/8oz

25g/1oz *Mu Erh* (wood ear fungus) or dried shiitake mushrooms

2 carrots, halved lengthwise

1 onion, quartered

1 fresh red chilli, washed but left whole

4 cloves garlic, left whole and unskinned

½ teaspoon black peppercorns

Pinch of salt

About 20g/¾oz piece of *Dang Gui*

About 20g/¾oz piece of *Dang Shen*

3 teaspoons cornflour

Fresh coriander leaves, to garnish

Clean and wash the pigeons. Place them whole in a large cooking pot and add the *Mu Erh* or shiitake mushrooms, carrot, onion, chilli, garlic, peppercorns, salt, *Dang Gui* and *Dang Shen*. Cover with water, bring to the boil, cover and simmer over a low heat for about 2 hours, until the pigeons are cooked and tender. Make sure the stew does not boil dry and add more water if necessary. Towards the end of cooking time make sure that you have roughly 450ml/16fl oz stock remaining.

Remove the birds from the pan, skin them, remove the breast meat in a whole piece, then set aside and keep warm. Discard the bones and remaining parts of the pigeons.

Strain the cooking liquid, pick out the *Mu Erh* pieces or shiitake and some of the peppercorns and discard the rest. Shred the cooked fungus or shiitake and return it to the stock with the reserved peppercorns. Squeeze the paste from the garlic cloves and add it to the stock.

Return the stock to the heat. Mix the cornflour with a little water and stir into the stock. Heat gently until the mixture has thickened to the consistency of a light sauce.

Adjust the seasoning if required, then return the pigeon breasts to the pan. Cook for a few minutes to warm them through. Arrange the pigeon breasts on a warm serving plate, pour over a little of the sauce, and garnish with coriander leaves. Serve with the remaining sauce and mashed potatoes.

Cinnamon Pancakes

Chinese cinnamon (*Rou Gui*) is a potent tonic for kidney *yang* which warms and strengthens kidney *Qi*. It is also traditionally regarded as a sexual tonic for both men and women. *Rou Gui* is much richer tasting than the culinary cinnamon commonly used in the West, so try to use the Chinese variety if you can in this recipe.

The cranberries are cleansing for the urinary system, so this dish will also be helpful to those with a tendency for problems such as cystitis.

Serves 4-6

For the topping:
175g/6oz fresh or frozen cranberries
225g/8oz clear honey or maple syrup
2 tablespoons orange juice

For the pancakes:
225g/8oz organic plain flour (brown or white)
115g/4oz soft brown sugar
1 teaspoon baking powder
½ teaspoon *Rou Gui*
Pinch of salt
275ml/½ pint cow's milk or soya milk
1 large egg
2-3 tablespoons olive oil

Start by making the cranberry and honey topping. Combine the cranberries, 175g/6oz honey or maple syrup and the orange juice in a small saucepan. Bring to the boil and simmer, uncovered, for 20 minutes. The berries will soften, colouring and flavouring the syrup.

Add the remaining honey or maple syrup and simmer for a further 5 minutes. Strain and discard the cranberries, reserving the syrup. Set aside and keep warm.

To make the pancakes, mix together the flour, sugar, baking powder, *Rou Gui* and salt. In another bowl, whisk together the milk and egg. Pour this mixture over the dry ingredients and whisk well.

Heat a frying pan, brush with a little oil, then ladle a little of the pancake mixture into the pan to form a thin coating. Fry for 2-3 minutes, then toss/turn the pancake and cook on the other side until golden. Keep the pancakes hot by stacking them on a plate set on top of a bowl of very hot water while you cook the rest.

Serve the pancakes with a little of the cranberry-flavoured syrup.

The cranberry topping will keep in a clean jar for 2 weeks in the refrigerator. Reheat before serving by heating the jar in a saucepan of hot water.

Rou Gui

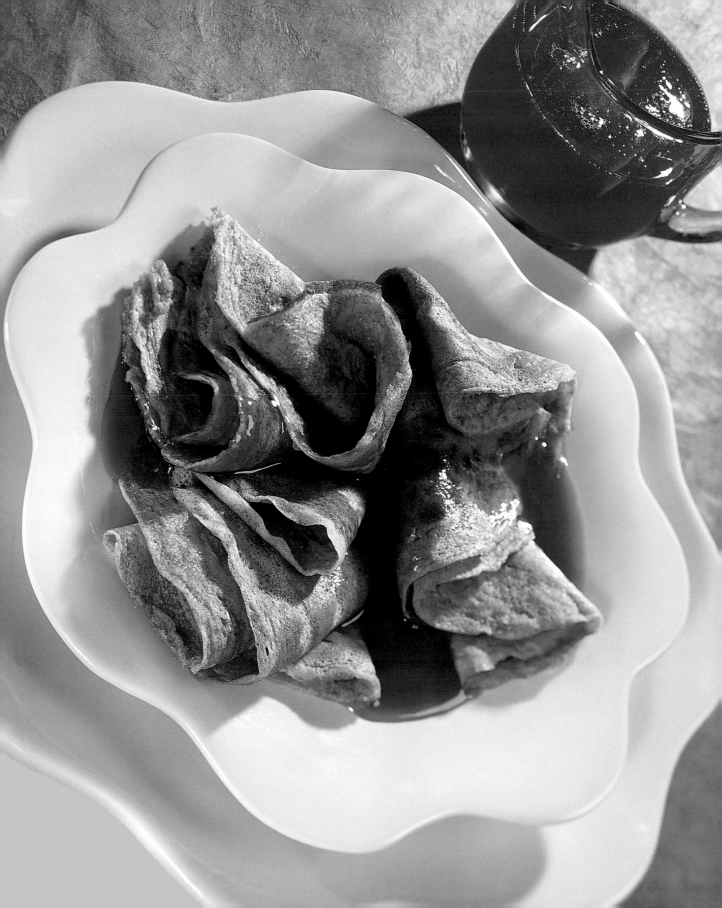

Nourishing Hidden Treasures Rice Pudding

This dish will nourish blood and kidney *Qi* so can be especially suitable for women suffering from "deficient blood" associated with menstrual irregularities, while the focus on kidney *Qi* makes it ideal at the menopause. The nuts used in this recipe are also a good source of essential fatty acids.

Sweet bean paste, made from red beans, is popular in China as a filling for steamed buns. It is available in Chinese food stores and can be stored in the refrigerator almost indefinitely.

Serves 6-8

570ml/1 pint cow's milk or soya milk
400g/14oz pudding rice
85g/3oz brown sugar
55g/2oz *Gou Qi Zi* (lycii berries), washed
55g/2oz *Long Yan Rou* (longan) washed
55g/2oz red and black dates (*Hong Zao* and *Da Zao*), washed and chopped
55g/2oz stem ginger, chopped
55g/2oz walnuts, chopped
55g/2oz pine nuts
55g/2oz whole almonds
85g/3oz sweet bean paste
Cream or crème fraîche, to serve (optional)

Put the milk and rice into a non-stick saucepan and bring the mixture to the boil. Simmer for 15 minutes or until most of the milk has been absorbed by the rice grains.

Drain the rice and stir in the sugar, then mix in the Chinese herbs, dates, ginger, nuts and sweet bean paste.

Generously butter a pudding bowl and spoon in the rice mixture. Cover with a piece of greaseproof paper pleated in the middle, tie down with string, then wrap in a pudding cloth. Steam the pudding for 1½ hours.

Remove from the heat and allow to cool slightly before turning out into a clean dish. Serve with cream or crème fraîche.

Sunflower and Sesame Spread

This combination of nuts and seeds will help lubricate the large intestine and is excellent for a sluggish digestion. It is an ideal spread for the sort of constipation common in old age and associated with weakened digestive energy.

Sesame seeds and pine nuts are soothing and lubricating for the lungs so the spread is also ideal for moistening a dry, irritant cough.

Serves about 8

55g/2oz pine nuts
55g/2oz white sesame seeds
55g/2oz walnuts
1 tablespoon maple syrup
4 tablespoons apple juice
Pinch of salt

Toast the pine nuts and sesame seeds in a dry, non-stick frying pan until they turn brown.

Put the toasted pine nuts and sesame seeds in a blender or food processor with the walnuts and blend until smooth.

Transfer to a mixing bowl and add the maple syrup, apple juice and salt, mixing well. Add a little water or more apple juice if the mixture seems too thick.

Spread on bread, rice cakes or oat cakes for a tea-time treat. Store in a jar or plastic pot with a lid and use as required.

Walnut and *Long Yan Rou* Chews

Walnuts strengthen and warm the kidneys helping to relieve problems such as impotence and lower back pain. They are warming and sweet, soothing and lubricating for the bowels and ideal for symptoms of "kidney yang deficiency" which can include coughs and asthma.

The *Long Yan Rou* (longan fruits) are also warming and sweet. They invigorate the heart and spleen and moisten all five *Zang* organs (see page 11) as well as nourishing blood and *Qi*. They are a useful herb for combating tiredness, ageing and insomnia.

These sweets are an ideal tea-time snack.

Makes about 16

25g/1oz *Long Yan Rou*
3 tablespoons olive oil
1 tablespoon maple syrup
115g/4oz unrefined brown sugar
85g/3oz chopped walnuts
2 eggs, beaten
55g/2oz desiccated coconut
115g/4oz plain white or wholemeal flour, sifted
1 teaspoon baking powder
Pinch of salt

Preheat the oven to 180°C/350°F/gas mark 4. Grease a shallow 20cm/8in square cake tin and set aside.

Rinse the *Long Yan Rou* in water and soak in fresh hot water for 10 minutes, then drain and chop finely.

Combine all the ingredients, including the *Long Yan Rou*, in a bowl and mix well. Transfer the mixture to the prepared tin and spread evenly.

Bake in the oven for 25 minutes until golden brown. Turn out onto a cooling rack, leave to cool, then cut into 5cm/2in squares. Serve cold.

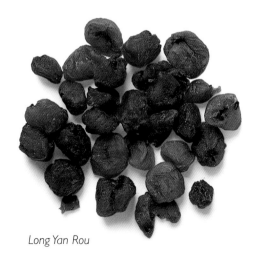

Long Yan Rou

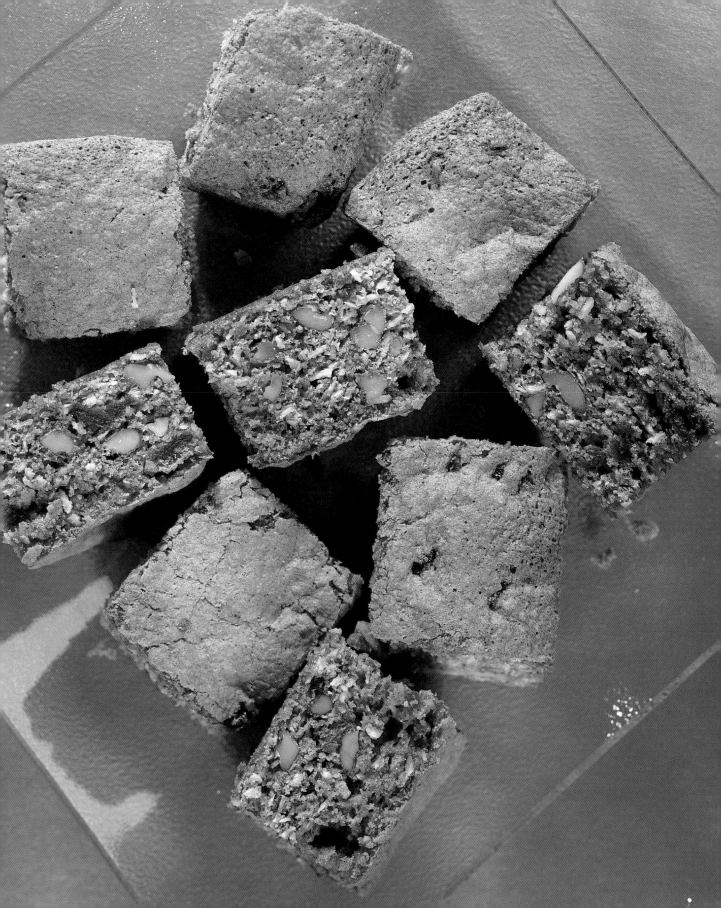

Ginger and Cinnamon Ice Cream

Traditionally, the Chinese do not eat cold foods such as ice cream, as they believe that these foods are damaging to the spleen, disturbing the digestive cauldron of the *San Jiao* (see page 105) and causing stagnation of food and reduced metabolism in the gut.

However, ginger and cinnamon are both warming for the digestion and together can help balance the cooling effect of ice-cream – they're good to eat at the same time.

Serves 4-6

280g/10oz jar stem ginger in syrup
8 organic egg yolks
115g/4oz refined cane sugar
570ml/1 pint milk
275ml/½ pint double cream
Finely grated zest of 1 orange
¼ teaspoon *Rou Gui* (cinnamon powder)

Chop all but 3 pieces of ginger in a blender or food processor. Set aside, reserving the syrup. Whisk the egg yolks and 55g/2oz sugar together in a bowl and set aside.

Put the milk, cream, orange zest, *Rou Gui*, ginger syrup (there should be about 120ml/4fl oz syrup left after draining the stem ginger) and the remaining sugar into a saucepan and bring just to the boil.

Pour half of this mixture onto the egg yolks and whisk gently together. Pour the egg mixture back into the pan and stir constantly over a gentle heat until the custard thickens enough to coat the back of a spoon, being extra careful not to overcook it.

Pour the thickened custard into a bowl and whisk in the chopped stem ginger. Leave to cool.

Put the mixture into an ice-cream maker, churn according to the manufacturer's instructions and freeze. Alternatively, put in the freezer in a shallow, freezer-proof container. When half frozen (after 1-2 hours), place the ice cream into the food processor and blend, then return to the container and freeze until firm.

Chop the 3 remaining pieces of ginger finely and use to decorate the scoops of ice cream.

What the Chinese categorise as damp and "phlegm" problems are especially common in Western society. "Damp" is one of the external evils which traditional Chinese medicine blames for superficial or external illness – disorders such as colds, minor infections or muscular aches and pains. "Phlegm" in TCM is rather different from our Western concept of a sort of catarrhal mucus produced during vigorous bouts of coughing.

The Chinese model has two sorts of phlegm – visible and invisible. The visible is our familiar sputum, but the invisible collects inside the body and can be both a cause and product of disease. Spleen *Qi* deficiency, for example, will lead to the production of phlegm, which will then move towards the heart causing a blockage.

Eating plenty of intrinsically sweet foods will help to restore balance to the system, but "sweet" does not mean the refined sugars associated with the word in the West: these simply increase dampness. "Sweet" foods include cooked carrots, sweet potatoes, turnips, leeks, onions, sweet rice, butter, lamb, chicken, cooked peaches, honey, maple syrup and unrefined sugars. Foods to avoid include salads, citrus fruit, salt, dairy products, refined sugars and too much liquid taken with meals.

Try some of these therapeutic dishes as well.

Clearing Damp and Phlegm

Aduki Bean Minestrone with *Chen Pi*

Aduki beans are considered the most digestible of all the beans used in Chinese cooking. They are neutral with a sweet and sour taste so are helpful for both spleen and liver. They also help to combat fluid retention and ease diarrhoea and liver stagnation.

In this recipe, they are combined with *Chen Pi* – mature tangerine peel – which is used in TCM to reverse the upward flow of *Qi*, associated with nausea, vomiting or profuse coughing.

Serves 4

115g/4oz dried aduki beans
10g/⅓oz *Chen Pi*
2 tablespoons olive oil
1 onion, finely chopped
2 sticks celery, chopped
2 cloves garlic, crushed
1.3 litres/2¼ pints chicken or
    vegetable stock
225g/8oz leeks, chopped
2 large carrots, chopped
450g/1lb tomatoes, chopped
1 dessertspoon tomato
    purée
2 bay leaves
2 tablespoons long-grain rice
Salt and freshly ground black
    pepper
115g/4oz peas or sweetcorn
2 courgettes, chopped
2 tablespoons chopped fresh
    parsley
A few sprigs of fresh basil,
    to garnish

Soak the aduki beans and the *Chen Pi* in water for 2-3 hours.

Heat the oil in a saucepan and sauté the onion, celery and garlic for 2-3 minutes until soft. Strain the beans and *Chen Pi* and add to the onion mixture. Pour over the stock and bring to the boil. Reduce immediately to a slow simmer, cover and cook for 1 hour.

Add all the vegetables (except the peas or sweetcorn and courgettes), tomato purée and bay leaves, cover and simmer for a further 30 minutes. Add the rice, season to taste with salt and pepper, cover and simmer for a further 30 minutes.

A few minutes before the end of the cooking time add the courgettes, peas or sweetcorn and parsley and simmer until the vegetables are tender. Serve garnished with basil.

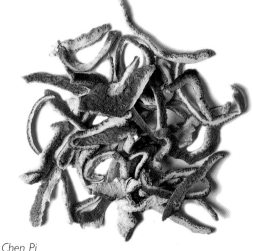

Chen Pi

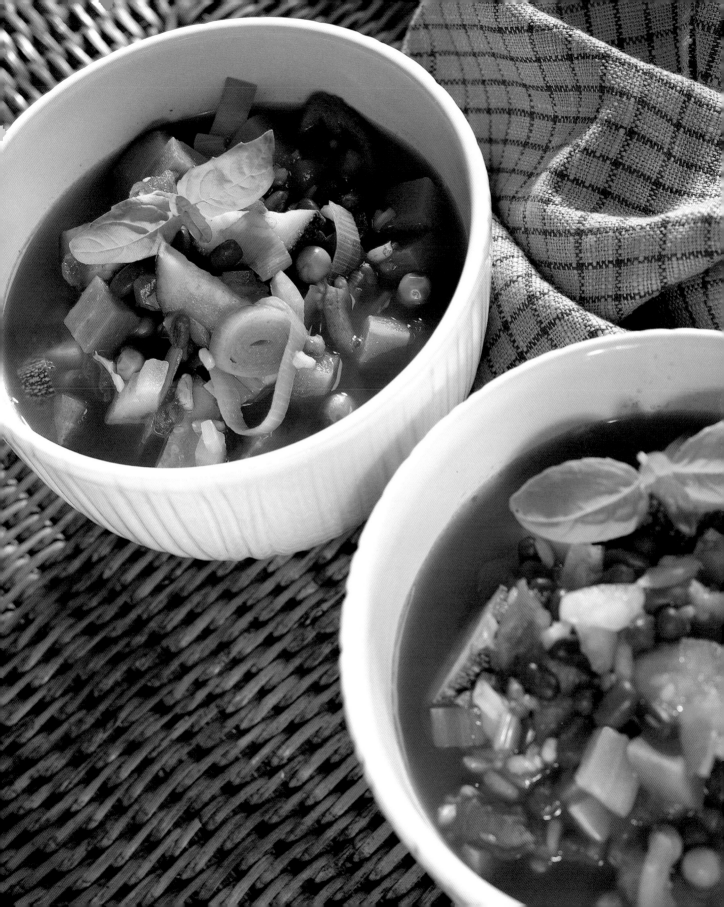

Smoked Eel and Watercress Salad

Eel (see page 172) is an excellent warming tonic for spleen and kidneys. In this recipe, it is combined with watercress *(Nasturtium officinale),* which is a pungent, bitter herb – stimulating for the digestion, diuretic and expectorant – also helps to clear dampness from the system. It is very rich in minerals and vitamins so is a good food in debility and convalescence as well. The horseradish *(Armoracia rusticana)* is also stimulating and warming, acting as a diuretic and improving circulation.

Serves 4 as a starter or 2 as a light lunch

350g/12oz smoked eel fillets

Juice of 1 lemon, plus 1 lemon slice per person, to garnish

4 tablespoons olive oil

1 tablespoon freshly grated horseradish

1 teaspoon Dijon mustard

Freshly ground black pepper

2 bunches watercress, washed well

Crème fraîche, to serve (optional)

Cut the eel fillets diagonally into strips and set aside. Whisk the lemon juice, oil, horseradish, mustard and pepper together.

Toss the watercress in the dressing and arrange on individual serving plates.

Sprinkle the eel slices over the watercress, add a lemon slice to garnish and serve with a spoonful of crème fraîche if you like.

Serve with chunks of French bread or ciabatta for lunch, or with thinner slices of rye bread for a light starter.

Beef Stir-Fry with *Chen Pi*

This warming dish, combining beef with garlic and ginger, helps to clear excess dampness, while the *Chen Pi* (tangerine peel) is a good tonic for the spleen and helps to regulate its action. "Deficient spleen or stomach *Qi*" or "spleen *yang* deficiency" are common causes of excess phlegm, with symptoms such as poor appetite, abdominal bloating and discomfort, tiredness and recurrent loose stools or diarrhoea. It is the sort of problem which might be labelled as "irritable bowel syndrome" in Western medicine and can also be associated with nervous indigestion or a tendency to gastric ulcers.

The sweeter tasting vegetables, such as carrots, also help the spleen. Swedes or sweet potatoes may be substituted if you prefer, although they need to be boiled for 15 minutes before being added to the stir-fry.

Serves 4

1 tablespoon *Chen Pi*
115g/4oz baby carrots,
 thinly sliced
115g/4oz baby leeks,
 washed and thinly sliced
1 dessertspoon olive oil
500g/1lb beef fillet, cut into
 thin strips
1 tablespoon seasoned plain
 flour
1 clove garlic, crushed
1 teaspoon peeled, chopped
 fresh root ginger
Pinch of granulated sugar
120ml/4fl oz rice wine or
 dry sherry
225ml/8fl oz vegetable, beef
 or chicken stock
1 heaped teaspoon
 arrowroot, stirred into a
 paste with a little water
Salt and freshly ground
 black pepper

Soak a piece of *Chen Pi* in a cup of boiling water for 5-10 minutes to soften, then drain and cut into very thin slices. If you do not have any *Chen Pi* you can use the fresh peel of a ripe tangerine (organically grown or unwaxed) instead.

Stir-fry the carrots and leeks in the oil in a pan or wok until they start to soften. Chinese therapeutic meals should be cooked with as little oil as possible – if you have a non-stick pan it is usually possible to dry-fry meats, although vegetables may need a little oil to improve the cooking.

Toss the beef slices in the seasoned flour, then add to the pan or wok with the garlic, ginger, *Chen Pi* and sugar. Stir-fry for about 5 minutes until the meat is browned, then add the rice wine or sherry and bubble vigorously for a couple of minutes.

Add the stock and arrowroot paste and stir until thickened. Bring to the boil. Season to taste with salt and pepper and serve on a bed of plain boiled rice.

Thin slices of lamb fillet may be used instead of beef, if you prefer.

Salmon and Wakame with Buckwheat Noodles

Wakame seaweed (readily available in supermarkets and Chinese stores) nourishes *yin* and helps to transform phlegm. Phlegm production is closely associated with the spleen's role in separating the clear and turbid fluids produced during digestion. Phlegm tends to be stored by the lungs – hence its physical manifestation in productive coughing. Asthma is also associated with excess phlegm, with the characteristic wheeziness described as the "sound of phlegm". Symptoms depend on where the phlegm is concentrated. If it is in the stomach it will lead to nausea and vomiting, if in the lung to coughing and shortness of breath, if in the heart to mental disturbances, coma or delirium and so on.

Wakame is also cooling for hot conditions. It is used here with warming herbs such as ginger and garlic.

Serves 2

2 fresh or dried shiitake mushrooms, sliced
2 pieces salmon fillet, each about 175g/6oz, skinned
1 teaspoon teriyaki sauce
5cm/2in piece fresh root ginger, peeled and finely chopped
2 spring onions, chopped
2 shallots, thinly sliced
2 cloves garlic, finely chopped
1 tablespoon sesame seed oil
2 teaspoons soy sauce
275ml/½ pint fish stock (see Basics, page 187)
25g/1oz dried wakame seaweed
1 teaspoon mirin
150g/5oz buckwheat noodles

If using dried shiitake, soak the mushrooms in warm water for 10-15 minutes before draining and slicing. Set aside.

Brush the salmon fillets with teriyaki sauce and cook under a preheated hot grill for 3-5 minutes on each side, or until cooked through (thicker pieces of fillet will take longer). Keep warm.

In a hot wok, stir-fry the ginger, spring onions, shallots and garlic in a little of the sesame oil for 2 minutes, then add the soy sauce. Remove from the wok and put to one side. Keep warm.

Stir-fry the shiitake in the remaining sesame oil for 1 minute, then remove from the wok and set aside. Add the fish stock to the wok and heat to just below boiling, then remove the wok from the heat and add the wakame and mirin.

Meanwhile, cook the buckwheat noodles in boiling water according to the instructions on the packet until tender, then drain.

Divide the noodles between 2 soup bowls and pour over the hot stock with the wakame. Top with the mushrooms and salmon fillets and finally garnish with the ginger and garlic. Serve immediately.

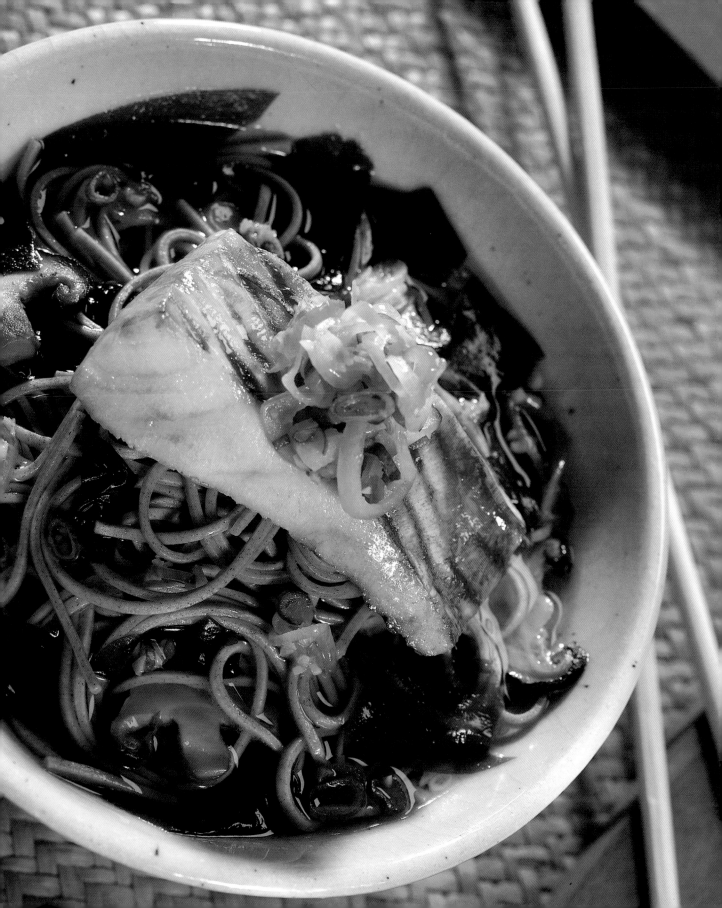

Buckwheat Noodle Soup with Purple Seaweed

Buckwheat *(Fagopyrum esculentum)* is cooling with a sweet flavour, it tonifies *Qi* and blood and clears heat. Buckwheat also stimulates the appetite and eases indigestion.

The Chinese purple seaweed is known as *nori* in Japan and is very similar to Welsh laverbread. It is cold, with a salty and sweet flavour. It also tonifies *Qi* and blood and is said to "transform phlegm and soften hardness" so is ideal for various damp conditions. Like other seaweeds, it is rich in iodine and was commonly used for thyroid problems like goitre.

This combination makes a delicious soup for stimulating the digestion and clearing excess phlegm.

Serves 4

- **1 litre/1¾ pints fish stock (see Basics, page 187)**
- **1 teaspoon finely grated peeled fresh root ginger or pickled ginger**
- **4 fresh oyster mushrooms, trimmed and sliced**
- **1 teaspoon mirin**
- **2 teaspoons shoyu soy sauce**
- **2 teaspoons Thai fish sauce or anchovy essence**
- **115g/4oz dried buckwheat (*somen*) noodles**
- **115g/4oz tofu, cut into small cubes**
- **115g/4oz mangetout, thinly sliced**
- **1 sheet of *nori* or 55g/2oz laverbread, cut into fine shreds**
- **2 spring onions, shredded**

Bring the fish stock to the boil in a pan, reduce to a simmer and add the ginger, mushrooms, mirin, shoyu, fish sauce or anchovy essence and buckwheat noodles. Stir over a low heat for 8 minutes.

Add the tofu, mangetout and *nori* or laverbread and simmer for a further 2 minutes.

Serve in soup bowls topped with the spring onions.

Thick Herby Leek Tart

Leeks are pungent and warming – regarded in China as a good *yang* food to help energise lungs and liver. They are traditionally eaten to clear cold, "excess stomach heat" and "stagnant blood" (see page 84), as well as calming *yin* and tonifying *Qi*.

They are important in Western tradition, too: used to clear phlegm in chesty coughs and to relieve ear-ache, as well as improving the eyesight. This last is a neat overlap with the Oriental association with the liver, which the Chinese also connect with vision and the eyes. Leeks can also be used, like onion, as a basis for cough mixtures and to help clear toxic wastes from the system.

Combined with stimulating Western herbs, this tart makes an ideal energising food.

Serves 6

For the pastry:
55g/2oz plain white flour
55g/2oz plain wholemeal flour
Pinch of salt
½ teaspoon baking powder
½ teaspoon mustard powder
85g/3oz butter, cubed

For the filling:
700g/1½lb leeks
55g/2oz butter
1 tablespoon chopped fresh oregano
2 teaspoons chopped fresh thyme
2 teaspoons very finely chopped fresh rosemary
Salt and freshly ground black pepper
3 eggs, beaten
115g/4oz natural yoghurt
1 tablespoon grated hard cheese such as Cheddar

Make the pastry by first sifting the flours, salt, baking powder and mustard powder into a bowl. Add the butter and rub together until the mixture has the consistency of breadcrumbs. Add 1-2 tablespoons water and knead to make a dough. Wrap in plastic film or a cloth and let the dough rest for at least 30 minutes in the refrigerator. Preheat the oven to 180°C/350°F/gas mark 4.

Trim and wash the leeks thoroughly (this is best done by slicing about 2.5cm/1in lengthwise through the top green part, then standing the leeks upside down in a beaker of water for a few minutes). Slice the white parts horizontally and the green sections lengthwise into ribbons.

Melt the butter in a large frying pan or wok and add the leeks. Stir well to coat with butter and then cook very gently for about 20 minutes until the leeks are soft and golden brown. Stir the herbs into the leek mixture and season to taste with salt and pepper.

Roll out the pastry and use it to line a greased 20cm/8in flan tin. Prick the base all over with a fork and bake blind for 15 minutes. Remove from the oven and brush the inside of the pastry case with a very little egg; then return to the oven and cook for a further 5 minutes.

Mix the remaining eggs with the yoghurt. Spread the leek and herb mixture over the base of the pastry case and pour over the egg and yoghurt mixture. Sprinkle the top with the grated cheese. Bake in the oven for about 30 minutes until golden and puffy. Serve warm or cold (though it is better warm) with salad or cooked green vegetables.

Steamed *Ge Gen* Dumplings Filled with Sweetened Pumpkin and *Shan Yao*

These dumplings are ideal to strengthen digestion and stimulate sluggish spleen energy.

Shan Yao (Chinese wild yam) is neutral with a sweet flavour. It is especially beneficial for the spleen, tonifies the lungs, reinforces the kidneys and replenishes *Jing* (vital essence). *Shan Yao* also helps encourage tissue growth. *Ge Gen* (kudzu) is cooling, mildly sweet and a little sour in flavour. It strengthens deficient spleen, associated with diarrhoea, and nourishes stomach fluids to relieve thirst.

Pumpkin is sweet and it also tonifies *Qi* and blood, dries damp and – like *Ge Gen* – encourages sweating, so is good in feverish conditions.

Makes about 24 dumplings

For the filling:
**55g/2oz brown or palm
  sugar**
**280g/10oz peeled and
  seeded pumpkin, cooked
  and mashed to a paste**
25g/1oz *Shan Yao* powder
85g/3oz tapioca flour
¼ teaspoon jasmine essence

For the dough:
115g/4oz gluten-free flour
**3 tablespoons powdered
  *Ge Gen***
Pinch of salt
**1 tablespoon olive or
  safflower oil**

Make the filling by dissolving the sugar in 1-2 tablespoons hot water in a bowl. Add all the remaining ingredients, mix well and set aside.

To make the dough, sift the flour and *Ge Gen* into a bowl, add the salt and oil, Pour over 170ml/6fl oz boiling water and whisk together. Set aside to cool.

When cool, knead until the dough is smooth. Divide into two long sausages about 2.5cm/1in in diameter. Wrap the dough rolls in plastic film to keep them moist.

When ready to use, cut each sausage into 1cm/½in slices and roll out each slice into a 10cm/4in diameter circle.

Place a spoonful of the filling in the centre of each dough round, moisten the edges of the dough with a little water and fold over the filling to make a bundle, pinching the edges together to seal. Place on greaseproof paper in a bamboo steamer and steam for 8-10 minutes.

Serve for breakfast or as *Dim Sum* – a light pre-lunch snack.

Ge Gen

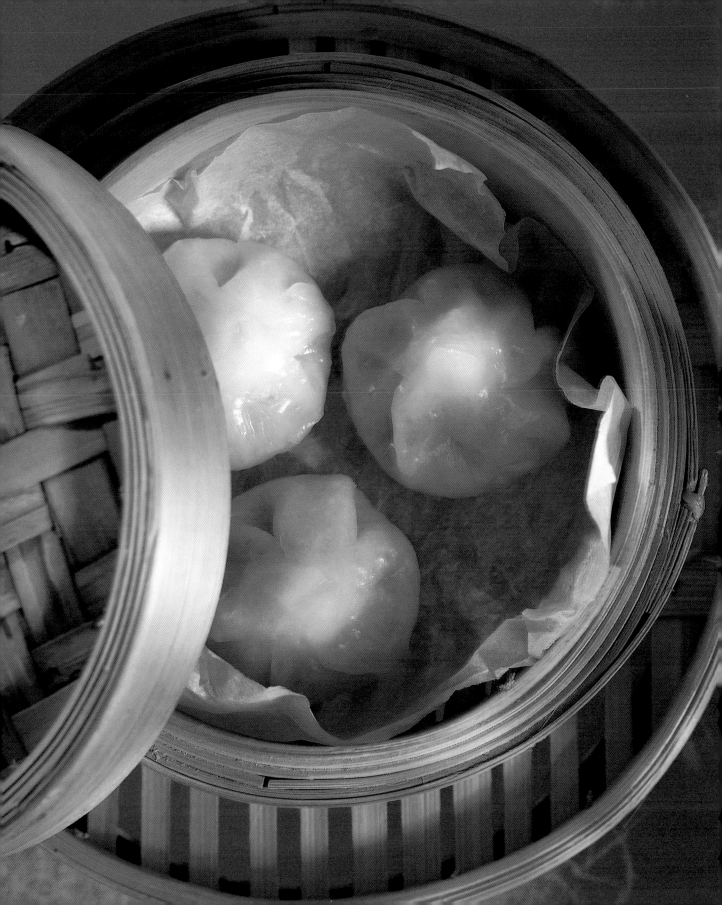

Eel Ease

Eel is warm with a sweet flavour. It is especially beneficial for liver, spleen and kidney, helping to strengthen muscles and bones, so it is a good food to eat regularly for arthritic and rheumatic conditions. Its tonifying action on the spleen makes eel an ideal food for clearing damp and phlegm. It is also a good *yang* food for spring.

In this recipe, the whole eel is roasted with garlic and parsley, which are both warming and helpful for the spleen. Fresh eel usually needs to be ordered from fish shops and it is best to ask the fishmonger to clean and skin the eel for you.

Serves 4

700g/1½lb fresh skinned eel
115g/4oz fresh parsley, chopped
Juice of 1 lemon
5 cloves garlic, crushed
200ml/7fl oz dry white wine
Sea salt
2 tablespoons olive oil

Preheat the oven to 190°C/375°F/gas mark 5. Make a series of shallow perpendicular cuts along the back of the cleaned eel. Prepare a marinade by mixing together half the parsley, the lemon juice, garlic and half the wine. Rub the eel all over with salt, then rub in some of the marinade and pour over the remainder.

Heat the olive oil in a round baking dish and spiral the eel into it pouring over the marinade. Roast in the oven for about 30 minutes, basting from time to time with the wine and oil mixture.

When the eel is cooked, it can be filleted and cut into portions. To fillet the eel, cut it along the backbone: start just behind the head, then turn the knife towards the tail and cut along the length of the eel against the backbone lifting the fillet as you go. Turn the eel over and repeat on the other side. Lift the second fillet clear of the spine.

Transfer the eel slices or fillets to a serving dish and sprinkle with the remaining wine and parsley. Serve with a green salad and boiled rice.

Poached Pears with *Chuan Bei Mu* and *Lian Zi*

Pears are cooling with a sweet flavour and have a special affinity for lungs and stomach. They are moistening, encouraging the production of body fluids *(Jin-Ye)*, as well as generally nourishing the lungs. They are an ideal food for coughs associated with heat and phlegm – productive coughs with infected phlegm such as in acute bronchitis and flu.

In this recipe, they are combined with *Chuan Bei Mu* (fritillary bulb) which helps to remove heat-phlegm from the lungs and relieve coughs or asthma. As well as helping specific lung problems, *Chuan Bei Mu* soothes the lungs and chest and restores a tired voice – ideal for singers or speakers!

Lian Zi (lotus seeds) are nourishing and cool, helping to support the action of the pears and *Chuan Bei Mu*.

Serves 4

15g/½oz Chuan Bei Mu
15g/½oz prepared or dried
   Lian Zi (see page 144)
4 firm ripe pears
175g/6oz unrefined sugar
225g/8oz can water
   chestnuts, drained or
   8 peeled fresh water
   chestnuts, left whole or
   halved
Candied orange peel, to
   decorate
Crème fraîche or cream,
   to serve (optional)

Simmer the *Chuan Bei Mu* in 450ml/16fl oz water for 30 minutes, then strain, reserving the liquid but discarding the herb.

If using dried *Lian Zi*, soak the seeds in water for 10 minutes, then drain. Peel and halve the pears and carefully remove the cores. Set aside.

Using a heavy-based pan, prepare the syrup by dissolving the sugar in the reserved fritillary bulb liquid over a low heat. Add the *Lian Zi* and water chestnuts and bring to the boil.

Carefully place the pears in the syrup and simmer for 10 minutes, gently turning over once during cooking.

Serve hot immediately, or remove the pears from the syrup to cool. When cool, return to the cooled syrup and serve cold. Decorate with candied orange peel.

It is best to avoid dairy products when suffering from excess mucus or phlegm – if this is not a problem, serve with crème fraîche or cream, if liked.

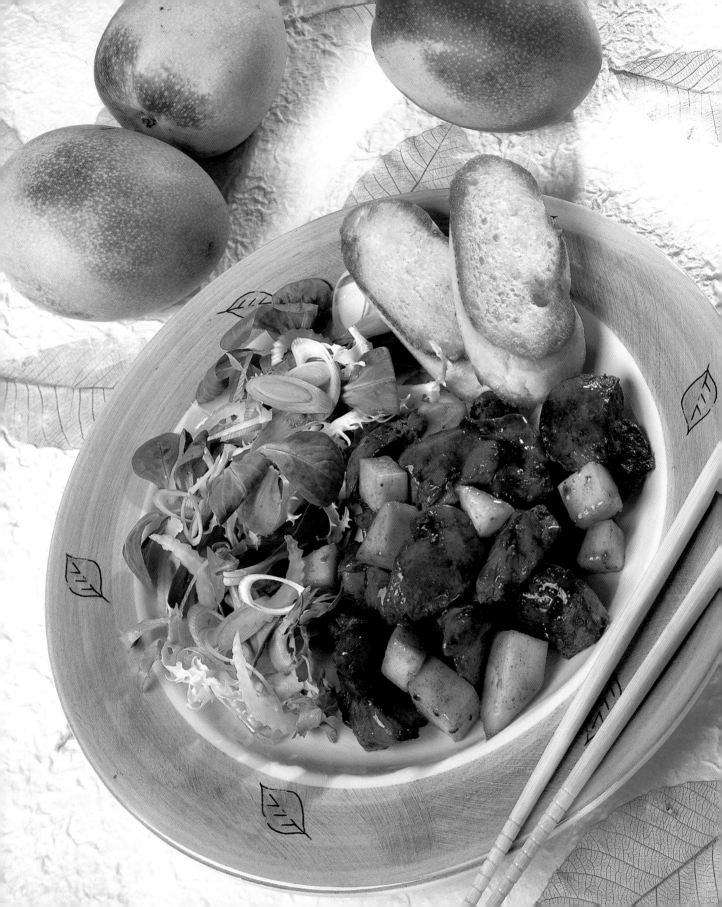

Problems associated with liver *Qi* imbalance are also common syndromes in the West. They are often typified by emotional instability – irritability or anger, a sensation of a lump in the throat or problems swallowing or lumps in the neck, groin or breast (including benign fibrocystitis).

Excess liver syndromes can include:
- "flaring liver fire" – usually associated with sore eyes, headaches, irritability, dizziness, nose bleeds and constipation;
- "over-exuberant liver *yang*" – headaches and sore eyes are likely to be accompanied by insomnia and palpitations;
- "liver *Qi* stagnation" – which is most commonly associated with menstrual irregularities.

Cooling *yin* remedies are often recommended for the first two categories with more stimulating liver tonics (see With Women in Mind, page 79) used for "liver *Qi* stagnation".

Typical Western disorders that may come into the "excess liver *Qi*" category include stress, abdominal bloating, irritable bowel syndrome, premenstrual syndrome, depression or period pain.

The liver is the body's first line of defence, taking the products of digestion, checking that they are not harmful and then adding them to the blood system. Toxic chemicals tend to remain "stuck" in the liver; Western herbalists, as well as Chinese ones, regularly talk of the "liver stagnation" which these pollutants cause.

Controlling Liver Qi

**Chicken livers and mango
(recipe on page 176)**

Chicken Livers and Mango

Chicken liver is a good relaxing food for the liver, helping to ease *Qi* stagnation. Spicy foods and herbs, such as black pepper, also help to activate and move *Qi*, although too much can be damaging.

Mango helps to lower excess liver *yang* and fire. Some other fruits, including peaches and plums, can also help to stimulate and cleanse the liver and may be substituted for mango in this recipe, if you like.

Serves 4

8 slices of French bread
3-4 tablespoons plus 1
  dessertspoon olive oil
450g/1lb fresh chicken livers,
  cut into bite-sized pieces
1-2 tablespoons seasoned
  plain flour
1 tablespoon balsamic
  vinegar
1 small ripe mango, peeled,
  stoned and cut into cubes
Pinch of granulated sugar
Salt and freshly ground black
  pepper

To make the croutons, fry the French bread in 3-4 tablespoons olive oil until crisp and golden. Set aside.

Toss the chicken livers in seasoned flour so that they are well coated. Stir-fry in the remaining oil for about 5 minutes, until they are browned on the outside but not overcooked.

Add the vinegar and let it bubble for 1 minute, then remove the pan from the heat, add the mango, sugar and salt and pepper and mix well.

Serve on a bed of lettuce with a little shredded celery and sliced baby leeks added, accompanied by the French bread croutons.

Tomato Soup with Dandelion

Tomatoes help to clear heat and strengthen *yin* while dandelion is a good liver decongestant. Dandelion root is more effective as a liver tonic than the leaves, so, if available, you can add 3-4 tablespoons of dandelion root decoction to the soup while it is simmering. This soup can be helpful for problems associated with liver *Qi* stagnation or excess liver *yang*.

Serves 4

1 onion, finely chopped
55g/2oz unsmoked streaky bacon, diced
1 tablespoon olive oil
225g/8oz potatoes, diced
450g/1lb tomatoes, skinned and coarsely chopped
1 tablespoon organic tomato purée
425ml/¾ pint chicken stock
Salt and freshly ground black pepper
Handful of fresh young dandelion leaves
Croutons or natural yoghurt and chopped fresh chives, to serve (optional)

Sauté the onion and bacon in the olive oil in a large saucepan for 2-3 minutes, then add the potatoes and cook for 1-2 minutes.

Add the tomatoes, tomato purée and stock, bring to the boil, cover and simmer for 25-30 minutes, until the mixture is soft and well blended.

Season to taste with salt and pepper and whisk thoroughly or purée in a blender or food processor to give a smoother soup. Return to the rinsed-out saucepan.

Wash and coarsely chop the dandelion leaves and stir into the soup. Return to the heat, bring to the boil and simmer for 5 minutes to reheat.

Serve with croutons or garnish with a little yoghurt and chives, if preferred.

Artichokes and Shiitake Mushrooms

Globe artichokes (*Cynara scolymus*) are not only good to eat, they are an extremely therapeutic herb – a bitter digestive remedy to stimulate and strengthen liver and gall bladder. Artichokes contain a substance called cynarin which is believed to enhance the liver's action in clearing toxins from the blood and to generally revitify its action; it also helps with fat metabolism, so can reduce high blood cholesterol levels. Studies also suggest that artichokes have a similar strengthening action on the kidneys.

In this recipe, they are combined with shiitake mushrooms which, as well as strengthening the immune system, have been shown to protect the liver, stimulate its function and combat certain types of hepatitis. The *Huang Qi* wine is also immune-stimulating.

Poor liver function is often associated with the signs of ageing as well as with such health problems as migraine, diarrhoea and constipation – so this recipe is ideal as a general liver tonic at any age.

Serves 4

6 large globe artichoke heads
4 tablespoons lemon juice
150g/5oz smoked lean back bacon, coarsely chopped
3 tablespoons extra-virgin olive oil
120ml/4fl oz *Huang Qi* wine (see page 184), or substitute dry white wine
225g/8oz fresh shiitake mushrooms, sliced
Salt and freshly ground black pepper
1 egg yolk
½ teaspoon cornflour

Trim and slice the artichokes, discarding the stalks, hairy chokes and tough leaves. Put them into a bowl of cold water with 2 tablespoons lemon juice, to prevent them from discolouring. Set aside.

Fry the bacon in the oil until crisp. Drain and dry the artichokes and add them to the frying pan. Cook for about 3 minutes, then pour in half the wine.

Add the shiitake mushrooms, season to taste with salt and pepper, then cover and cook for about 10 minutes.

Mix the egg yolk with the cornflour in a basin, then add the remaining lemon juice and wine and stir until well blended.

Pour this over the artichoke mixture and stir constantly over a very low heat until the sauce thickens. Serve with boiled new potatoes or Herby Mash Potatoes (see page 104).

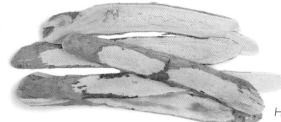

Huang Qi

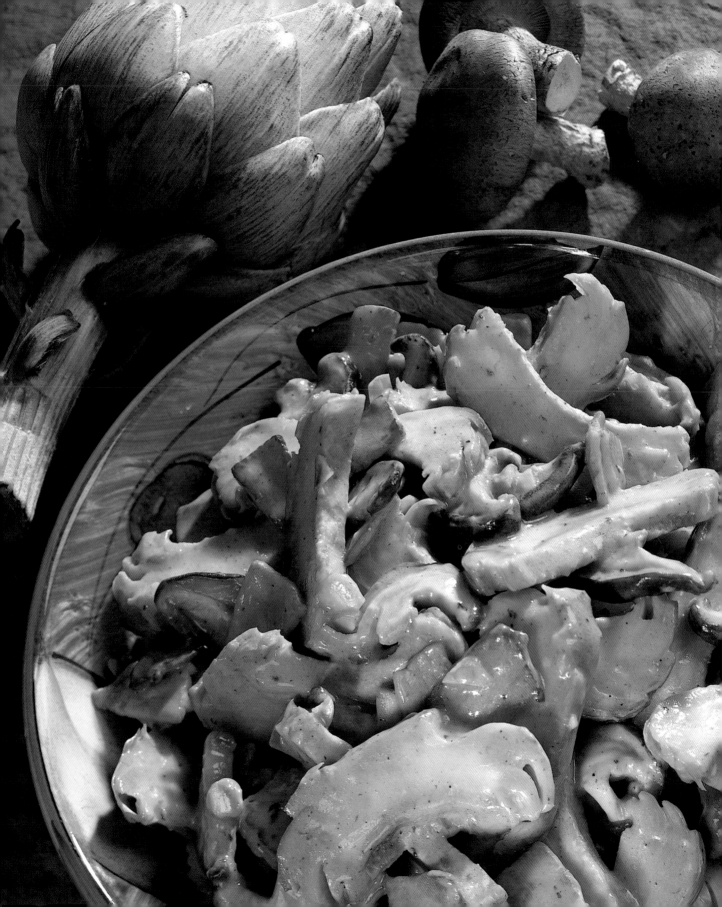

Ju Hua and *Jin Yin Hua* Sorbet

Ju Hua (chrysanthemum flowers) are slightly cold with a mixed pungent, sweet and bitter flavour. They act specifically on the liver and lung channels and will clear wind, heat and toxins. They are an important remedy in Chinese medicine for problems associated with "hyperactivity of liver *yang*" – typified by headaches and dizziness – and problems affecting the eyes (such as conjunctivitis) which are closely associated with excess or "ascending liver fire".

Jin Yin Hua (honeysuckle flowers) are cool and sweet; they also dispel heat and wind and clear toxins. The flowers are mainly used to reduce fevers and heal inflamed or pus-filled wounds.

Together these flowers will lower blood pressure, while chrysanthemum also helps fat metabolism and honeysuckle reduces cholesterol levels.

Serves 4-6
1 tablespoon *Jin Yin Hua*
6 flowerheads *Ju Hua*
200g/7oz granulated sugar
Juice of 2 lemons

Put the *Jin Yin Hua* and *Ju Hua* into a basin. Bring 570ml/1 pint water to the boil and pour over the flowers. Leave to infuse for 10 minutes. Strain through a sieve over a saucepan, keeping the tea and discarding the flower heads.

Add the sugar and lemon juice to the tea and stir over a gentle heat until the sugar has fully dissolved.

Pour into a bowl and allow to cool, then freeze in a shallow freezer-proof container. Before the mixture is set (after 1-2 hours), remove it from the freezer and whisk thoroughly, then return it to the freezer until firm. Alternatively, churn and freeze the sorbet mixture in an ice-cream maker, following the manufacturer's instructions.

Depending on your taste preference, you can add more or fewer flowerheads to make a stronger or weaker-tasting sorbet.

Tonic wines – known as *Jiu* – in China are a traditional and easy way to make and take healing herbs. Many use a single herb, although various combinations aimed at specific organs and energy problems have been developed over the centuries. These herbal wines can also be added, like brandy or vermouth, in cooking to provide flavour.

Alcoholic extraction has been used for making therapeutic tinctures, to obtain the active constituents of the plant in an easy-to-use form, for at least 2000 years. Alcohol also acts as a preservative, so these tinctures generally last for at least two years without significant deterioration.

Small amounts of alcohol will supplement and move *Qi* and vitalise the spirit, although larger quantities will have the opposite effect. Large amounts of alcohol are toxic, injuring body and mind. When used in cooking, the alcohol is partially evaporated by heat but the flavour stays.

Therapeutic Drinks

Walnut Vodka

As well as strengthening kidneys and lungs and nurturing essence (*Jing*) – see also page 12 – walnuts help to keep our skin smooth and moist and muscles well-toned. In Western tradition, they are considered an excellent food for the brain – a relic of the mediaeval Doctrine of Signatures, whereby a plant's appearance suggested its therapeutic actions: wrinkled walnut kernels reminded our ancestors of the brain.

Vodka is used in this recipe as its bland taste does not interfere with the walnut aroma, but brandy is just as suitable.

Walnut vodka can be used to flavour fruit salads, salad dressings, fruit cakes, desserts, meat marinades or just simply served as a drink.

200g/7oz fresh, good-quality walnuts
570ml/1 pint vodka

Chop the walnuts and put them in a glass jar. Cover with vodka and seal. Leave the jar to stand in a dark cabinet for 1 month and shake it occasionally.

Decant the fluid and store it in an airtight glass bottle.

The walnut dregs can be further used in fruit salads, crushed into salad dressings or simply added to a fruit cake mixture.

After-Dinner Red Date Brandy

The sweetness of red dates dissolved in brandy makes an interesting after-dinner drink, which also helps a weak stomach to digest heavy meals. The dates, discarded when the brandy is decanted, can be used in fruit cakes (after removing the stones) or chopped finely and added to fruit salads or meat dishes.

200g/7oz Chinese red dates (*Hong Zao*)
570ml/1 pint brandy

Make sure that the dates are clean (rinse and dry them if necessary). Place them in a glass jar, cover with brandy and seal.

Leave to stand for 1 month, shaking the jar every few days. Strain the fluid and store it in a sealed glass bottle.

Hui Shiang Jiu

Fennel (*Hui Shiang*) is an excellent herb for the digestion and for preventing food stagnation. It is prescribed in cases of lower abdominal pain associated with cold, poor appetite, abdominal distention and testicular pain.

115g/4oz *Hui Shiang* seeds
570ml/1 pint rice wine

Stir-fry the seeds quickly (without oil) in a thick-based frying pan for 1-2 minutes. Remove the pan from the heat, allow the seeds to cool slightly, then put them into a self-sealing glass preserving jar.

Add the rice wine, seal the jar and place it in a pan of water. Bring to the boil. Once the water starts boiling, reduce the heat. When it has gone off the boil, raise the heat again, bring the water back to boiling point, then reduce the heat again. Repeat this process once more, then turn off the heat and leave the jar to cool down in the saucepan of water.

When cool, decant the wine into a clean glass bottle and it is ready for use.

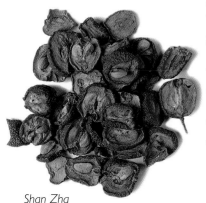

Shan Zha

Shan Zha Jiu

Shan Zha (Chinese hawthorn berries) are much larger fruits than the European species and have slightly different therapeutic properties. They are used mainly for digestive problems, whereas the European berries are more commonly associated with blood pressure remedies.

This wine promotes digestion, disperses stagnant food and eases abdominal bloating. It is ideal added as a dressing to any fruit salads, to make a therapeutic dessert following a large meal.

115g/4oz *Shan Zha*
115g/4oz Chinese red dates
(*Hong Zao*)
Generous pinch of *Rou Gui*
(powdered cinnamon)
25g/1oz soft brown sugar
1 litre/1¾ pints rice wine

Chop the *Shan Zha* and dates in a blender or food processor, then add the *Rou Gui* and sugar. Transfer the mixture to a glass jar and cover with the rice wine. Seal the jar and let it stand for 10 days, shaking it occasionally.

Decant the wine into a clean glass bottle through a jelly bag to remove the dregs. Seal and store for use.

Xi Yang Shen Wine

Xi Yang Shen (American ginseng) is sweet, slightly bitter and cool. It helps to strengthen *Qi,* nourish *yin* and generate fluids. *Xi Yang Shen* wine is ideal to help recovery from feverish illnesses or for throat problems and coughs. As well as making a delicious aperitif, this wine can be used for all sorts of meat marinades, especially duck, chicken and pigeon.

25g/1oz *Xi Yang Shen*
570ml/1 pint rice wine

Whole *Xi Yang Shen* roots need to be sliced into thin rounds. Place the *Xi Yang Shen* in a clean glass bottle, cover with the rice wine, seal the jar and leave to stand for a minimum of 2 weeks.

Keep the root in the bottle as long as the wine is at the level to cover it entirely and simply pour off the liquid as required.

Alternatively, use a vinegar vat – a crock pot holding 2-3 litres/3½-5¼ pints with an open top, closed with a large cork and a small tap at the bottom end. These can usually be bought in good-quality cookshops, from home wine-making specialists or from craft potters.

If using a vat put 225g/8oz *Xi Yang Shen* into the pot and cover with 3 litres/5 pints rice wine. Draw glasses of wine as required. The vat can be topped up with fresh wine and used for many months.

Huang Qi Jiu

Huang Qi (see page 69) is one of China's most stimulating tonic herbs. This wine is especially useful for those suffering from any weakness in the limbs, shortness of breath, or palpitations and sweating associated with *Qi* deficiency. It can be served as an aperitif to stimulate energy and strengthen the digestion.

115g/4oz *Huang Qi*
500ml/1 pint rice wine

Huang Qi is usually sold in shavings or thin sticks. Place the *Huang Qi* into a glass jar and cover with the rice wine. Seal the jar and leave it for 1 month, shaking the contents occasionally.

After a month, open the jar and strain the wine into a clean glass bottle. Seal. Serve in small schnapps glasses.

Dang Gui Jui

Dang Gui (Chinese angelica) is known in China as a woman's best friend: it is helpful for regulating menstruation and especially good in cases of painful or irregular menstrual flow. A tablespoon of the wine in a little water is ideal to relieve period pain. It is also good added to marinades.

115g/4oz *Dang Gui* (buy it sliced rather than a whole root)
570ml/1 pint brandy

Make sure the root is clean and dry, then place it in a glass jar, cover with brandy and seal. Leave to stand for about 1 month, shaking occasionally. Pour the fluid from the jar as required for as long as the herb is covered with brandy, then remove and discard the herb, or it will go mouldy.

Eye-Brightening Wine

Gou Qi Zi (lycii berries) – also known as the fruit of the matrimony vine – traditionally said to nourish the liver and kidney, benefit *Jing* and brighten the eyes. The sweet taste and rich colour of this wine enhance many dishes: it can be added to fruit salads, meat marinades and sauces.

115g/4oz *Gou Qi Zi*, washed
570ml/1 pint rice wine

Place the clean *Gou Qi Zi* in a glass jar and cover with rice wine. Seal the jar and leave to stand for about 2 weeks. Strain through a muslin bag and decant into a clean glass bottle. Seal. It is best to drink this wine by taking a dessertspoon in a cup of hot water in the morning.

Spice Rack Tea for Inner Clarity

Herbs affect more than just our physical well-being – many help to improve mental awareness and provide spiritual insights. The kitchen spice rack is full of suitable ingredients. Nutmeg in small amounts is calming for the mind. Liquorice root nourishes the lungs, reproductive, digestive and nervous systems. It has strong rejuvenating properties. Black cumin enhances the memory. Green cardamom stimulates the mind and heart and gives clarity and joy. It also increases perception, intelligence and harmony. Lemongrass relieves anxiety and has a slightly sedative effect.

Few grains grated nutmeg
Small liquorice stick
6 black cumin seeds
3 pods green cardamom
Shavings of lemongrass

Boil a mugful of water in a pan and add the nutmeg, liquorice, black cumin, cardamom and a few shavings of lemongrass. Cover and let it all simmer for 5 minutes, then strain into a mug and drink.

Karkade

In the Middle East, travellers are often welcomed with a glass of karkade, a tea made from hibiscus flowers which are cooling and cleansing in hot climates. In India, the hibiscus is sacred to the elephant god, Ganesh. Traditionally, karkade is served ice cold, but it also makes a pleasant hot drink in winter.

55g/2oz dried hibiscus petals
25g/1oz granulated sugar or clear honey

Soak the petals in 1 litre/1¾ pints cold water for 1-2 hours, then heat the mixture to boiling point. Strain, reserving the liquid, and return the petals to the pan, adding a fresh 1 litre/1¾ pints water. Bring to the boil again. Strain, reserving the liquid and discarding the petals. Combine the two batches of liquid, adding sugar or honey while the mixture is still hot.

Anti-Ageing Syrup

Huang Qi, ginseng and sage — along with *amachazuru* (see page 148) — are all established anti-ageing herbs. *Huang Qi* is a popular tonic in the East used to energise the whole body. Ginseng traditionally benefits all the *Qi* of the body, so that one may live a long and happy life. Sage has been extensively studied in Europe and is known to slow the progress of Alzheimer's disease and act as a powerful anti-oxidant to combat cell ageing. *Xi Yang Shen* (American ginseng) is more *yin* in character. It replenishes moisture and *Qi* and helps to balance the more heating *yang* energies of *Huang Qi* and Korean ginseng. *Amachazuru* could be added to the mixture instead of *Huang Qi* or ginseng.. The overall effect of these herbs enhances life energy, delays ageing, increases immunity and libido.

10g/⅓oz *Huang Qi*
10g/⅓oz Korean ginseng root
10g/⅓oz dried sage
10g/⅓oz *Xi Yang Shen*
310g/11oz granulated sugar

Place the herbs in a pan and pour over 570ml/1 pint water. Bring to the boil, cover and simmer for 1 hour to make a decoction. Strain into a measuring jug and discard the herbs, keeping the ginseng to chew on. Measure the decoction and make back up to 570ml/1 pint with water. Pour into the pan, add the sugar and heat gently, stirring, until the sugar has dissolved. Bring to the boil and boil for 10 minutes. Cool before bottling in a sterilised bottle. Seal with a cork, not a screwtop as syrups can ferment in storage and a tightly closed bottle might explode.

A daily dose (1 tablespoon) of this syrup should be used either poured over fruits or ice cream or as a concentrate for drinks. Try diluting it with ginger ale or fizzy water and serve with a slice of lemon as a restoring drink. When making syrups, make sure that the ratio of 65 per cent sugar to water is maintained.

Basics

Stocks

Many of the recipes in this book use vegetable or chicken-based stock. It is always best to prepare your own. Home-made stocks are low in salt and can be made in larger batches and then frozen; where possible use organic produce. All the stock recipes given here make 1½-2 litres/2¾-3½ pints

Vegetable Stock

2 large carrots, sliced
1 onion, sliced
3cm/1¼in piece fresh root
ginger, peeled and chopped
3 sticks celery, sliced
2 leeks, washed and sliced
1 courgette, sliced
2 cloves garlic, crushed

Mix all the ingredients in a large saucepan. Add 2 litres/3½ pints water, bring to the boil, cover and simmer for 2 hours. Strain, reserving the broth and discarding the vegetables.

The stock may be varied according to taste: try adding 1 tablespoon sesame seed oil, 1 table-spoon soy sauce, 2 chopped beetroots, 1 chopped parsnip or 5 fresh coriander stalks to the vegetables before adding the water. This stock can be kept for up to 3 days in the refrigerator or 3 months in the freezer.

Chicken Stock

Chicken bones are rich in marrow, which nourishes blood and essence (*Jing*).

1.5kg/3½lb chicken bones or
1 small whole chicken
3 sticks celery, sliced
1 onion, chopped
2 carrots, sliced
2 cloves garlic, crushed
1 leek, washed and sliced
5 fresh coriander stalks
1 thumb-sized piece fresh root ginger, peeled and chopped

Simmer the chicken, vegetables and herbs in 2½ litres/4 pints water in a large pot or slow cooker, covered, for 4 hours. Strain. When the stock has cooled, remove the fat.

The stock can be kept for up to 5 days in the refrigerator or 3 months in the freezer.

Fish Stock

1 fish, such as red mullet, about 225g/8oz in weight, gutted
Bunch each of fresh coriander, watercress and parsley
1 thumb-sized piece fresh root ginger, peeled and chopped

Put all the ingredients in a pan and add enough water to cover. Bring to the boil, then reduce the heat, cover and simmer for 2 hours. Skim any scum from the stock while it is simmering. Strain.

Cool, refrigerate and use within 24 hours or freeze for up to 3 months.

Herbal Mustards

Mixing herbs with mustard not only makes a convenient ready-to-use flavouring, but is an ideal way of preserving the summer's herb crop. This method works well with dill (leaves not seeds), coriander leaves, tarragon and basil.

2-4 tablespoons fresh herb
2-4 tablespoons Dijon mustard

Chop the herb in a small food processor. Add a roughly equivalent amount of Dijon mustard and then process to a well-blended paste. Store in a small sterile screw-top jar with greaseproof paper between the lid and the jar. This mustard will keep for 12-18 months in a refrigerator.

Aromatic Oils

Oil infusions are a versatile and convenient way of preserving the flavour of both fresh and dried herbs and spices. Good-quality olive oil with a lighter taste should be used. Avoid cold-pressed extra-virgin oil because of its strong flavour.

Both fresh herbs and dried spices can be made into aromatic oils by warm infusion. First, make sure that the herbs or spices are clean. If they need to be washed, pat them with a clean cloth or kitchen paper and air-dry them before proceeding further.

Put the prepared herb or spice into a preserving jar and cover with olive oil which has been gently heated to 30°C/86°F. Close the jar and place it on a cloth in the middle of the oven. Turn the oven on to its lowest setting and leave the oil to infuse there for 1 hour. Switch off the oven and leave the jar inside to cool down.

Strain the oil and herb or spice mixture into a preheated bowl through 4 layers of cheesecloth. Pour the oil into a sterilised jar or bottle, seal tightly, refrigerate and use within 2 weeks for the best flavour.

The following oils can be made by this method, using ½ cup of fresh herb to 250ml/½ pint olive oil:
• coriander oil
• basil oil
• rosemary oil
• oregano oil

Use the same method and ¼ cup dried herbs or spices to 250ml/½ pint olive oil for:
• ginger oil
• black pepper oil
• cinnamon oil
• star anise oil
• *Wu Wei Zi* oil
• *Dang Gui* oil

Black Cumin Oil

Use the method described above, but dry-roast the black cumin seeds first for 2-3 minutes in a thick-based pan. Use 1 cup black cumin seeds to 250ml/½ pint olive oil.

Safflower (Hong Hua) Oil

Safflower oil is commercially available and has a delicate taste with light texture. In order to turn the oil a deep saffron colour add ¼ cup safflower flowers and use the method described above.

Chilli Oil

4 fresh hot chillies or 8 dried hot chillies
275ml/½ pint olive oil

Remove and discard the seeds from the chillies, then chop the flesh finely in a food processor. Place in a pan with the oil and heat until the mixture begins to bubble. Let it cook for 10-15 seconds and then remove from the heat.

Swirl the pan contents until just warm, then strain into a hot bowl through 4 layers of cheesecloth. Pour the oil into a sterilised jar or bottle, seal tightly, cool, refrigerate and use within 2 weeks for the best flavour.

Garlic Oil

1 head raw garlic
120ml/4fl oz white vinegar
275ml/½ pint olive oil

Peel the garlic cloves and soak them in the vinegar for 15 minutes. Strain and rinse them under running water. Pat dry. Discard the vinegar.

Pour the oil into a glass jar with a stopper. Press the garlic through a garlic press into the oil, close the jar and shake gently for a few minutes. Leave to stand for 1 hour.

Strain through a fine mesh strainer, then through 4 layers of cheesecloth. Pour into a sterilised glass bottle. Close tightly, seal and refrigerate. Use within 1 week for optimum flavour.

Citrus-Flavoured Oils

It is important to look for fruit with a thin skin, since a large quantity of pith will make the oil bitter. Unwaxed,

organic fruit is also best – otherwise pesticide residues will be included on the skins.

Wash and dry the fruit thoroughly. Chop the fruit into thin pieces, transfer to the bowl of an electric mixer and add the oil. Using a paddle attachment, mix at a low speed for about 12 minutes. Stand at room temperature for about 2 hours.

Strain the contents through a fine mesh strainer, then through 4 layers of cheesecloth. Let the filtered liquid stand for long enough for the juice and oil to separate. The clear oil will float on top. Pour it carefully off into a sterilised glass jar or bottle. Cover tightly and refrigerate. Use within 1 week.

The following fruit oils can be made by this method. To 250ml/ ½ pint olive oil, add:
• 2 medium oranges
• 3 lemons
• 3 limes
• 300g/10oz kumquats
• 4 tangerines

Aromatic Vinegars

Vinegars can be made from red or white wine, cider, apples or other fruits and malted grains such as millet, barley, rice, wheat, etc. Vinegar is warming, sour and bitter and particularly affects the stomach and liver meridians. It also clears toxins, can disperse "blood stagnation" and stops nosebleeds.

Wine vinegars are produced from both red and white wines. The quality of vinegar depends on the quality of the wine used and the method of fermentation, as well as the quality of the wooden casks in which the vinegar is aged.

Champagne and sherry vinegars are also available and have a mellow, well-rounded flavour.

Rosemary, sweet rose petals, nasturtium flowers, citrus peel, tarragon, garlic, thyme, bay leaves, chives, spring onions and cinnamon are all ideal for flavouring vinegars. Fruits such as cherries, raspberries, bilberries, cranberries and elderberries may also be used.

Vinegars may be added to salad dressings, fruit salads, mayonnaise, fish dishes, pasta dressings, sauces and meat marinades. For oriental dishes, choose rice vinegar as the base: Japanese rice vinegars are mild, mellow and best flavoured with ginger, horseradish, mustard or lemongrass.

A vinegar vat (see page 184) is ideal for making a large quantity of vinegar. Otherwise use a glass preserving jar with a self-seal lid.

Herb or Spice Vinegars

115g/4oz fresh clean herb or spice
570ml/1 pint vinegar

Put the herb or spice into a vinegar vat or jar. Bring the vinegar to the boil and pour over the herb. Cover and seal the jar. Leave to infuse for 3 weeks, shaking occasionally.

Strain the vinegar into a sterilised glass bottle and cork tightly. The cork must first be sterilised by boiling for a few minutes in a pan of water.

Store in a cool, dark place. A low temperature is important for maintaining the flavour as well as the stability of home-made flavoured vinegar.

Fruit-Flavoured Vinegars

White wine vinegar is the best base for fruit flavouring as it allows the colour of the fruit to develop.

225g/8oz fruit – berries such as raspberries, wild blueberries, elderberries, blackcurrants or redcurrants are best
1 litre/1¾ pints white vinegar
1 tablespoon sugar

Prepare the fruit by removing all the green parts. If it needs to be washed, drip-dry in a muslin bag.

Use a glass preserving jar with a self-seal lid as before. Put the fruit into the jar and cover with the vinegar. Cover and leave to infuse for 2-3 weeks in a warm place, shaking the jar occasionally.

Strain the vinegar into a saucepan, add the sugar, stir and bring to the boil. Simmer gently for 10 minutes. Cool and pour into a sterilised jar. Seal and store.

Useful Addresses

Almost every large town now has shops selling Chinese ingredients in general and Chinese herbs in particular. Some of the largest are:

HAS International Foods,
189 Ormeau Road, Belfast BT7 1SQ

Wing Yip, 375 Nechells Park Road, Nechells, Birmingham B7 5NT

Janson Hong, St Martins House,
17/18 Bull Ring, Birmingham B5 5DD

Global Foods, Stadium Close,
Cardiff CF1 7TS

Chinaco, 67 Bride Street (off Camden Street), Dublin

Pats Chung Ying, 199 Leith Walk, Edinburgh EH6 8NX

Hongs, 7A Bath Street, Glasgow G2 1AA

Wing Lee Hong, 6 Edward Street, Leeds LS2 7NN

Chung Wah, 31/32 Great George Square, Liverpool L1 5DZ

Hondo, 5-11 Upper Duke Street, Liverpool L1 9DU

East/West Herbs, 3 Neals Yard, London WC2H

Neals Yard Remedies, 15 Neals Yard, London WC2H

Neals Yard Remedies, 68 Chalk Farm Road, London NW1

Neals Yard Remedies, 12 Chelsea Farmers Market, London SW3

Neals Yard Remedies, 9 Elgin Crescent, London W11

Wing Yip, 395 Edgware Road, Cricklewood, London NW2 6LN

Wing Yip, 544 Purley Way, Croydon CR0 4NZ

Loon Fung, 42-44 Gerrard Street, London W1V 7LP

Loon Moon, 9A Gerrard Street, London W1V 7LJ

See Woo Supermarket, 18-20 Lisle Street, London WC2

Hoo Hing, A406 North Circular Road, Near Hanger Lane, London NW10

Wing Yip, Oldham Road, Ancoats, Manchester M4 5HU

Wing Fat, 49 Faulkner Street, Manchester M1 4EE

Eastern Pearl, 27/31 Fenkle Street, Newcastle-upon-Tyne NE1 5XN

Lung Wah Cong, 41/42 Hythe Bridge Street, Oxford OX1 2EP

Sun Hung Chan, 6 Tricorn Shopping Centre, Portsmouth PO1 4AE

If none of these is convenient to you, or if they are unable to supply your needs, the following companies provide mail order services:

Acumedic Modern Chinese Healthcare, 101/105 Camden High Street, London NW1 7JN

East/West Herbs, 3 Neals Yard, London WC2H (small quantities only; wholesale orders to Langston Priory Mews, Kingham, Oxon OX7 6UW)

Neals Yard Remedies, Head Office 26-34 Ingate Place, London SW8 3NS

Hambledon Herbs, Court Farm, Milverton, Somerset TA4 1NF

Gourmet Mushrooms, Morants Farm, Colchester Road, Great Bromley, Colchester, Essex CO7 7TN

AUSTRALIA
MediHerb Pty PO Box 713, Warwick, Queensland 4370 (mostly supply professionals but stock some Chinese herbs),

Blackmores Ltd, 23 Roseberry Street, Balgowlah, NSW 2093

Greenridge Botanicals, PO Box1197, Toowoomba, Queensland 4350

Herbs of Gold Pty, 120 Millwood Avenue, Chatswood, NSW 2067

Nature's Sunshine Products of Australia Pty Ltd, Norwest Business Park, 19 Brookhollow Avenue, Baulkham Hills, NSW 2153

Phyto Pharmaceutical Products Pty Ltd, Unit 5, 2 Liverpool Street, Ingleburn, NSW 2565

Southern Light Herbs, 8 Sandy Creek Road, Maldon, Victoria 3463

CANADA
Gaia Garden Herbal Apothecary, 2672 W. Broadway, Vancouver, BC V6K 2G3

Richters Herbs, 357 Highway 47, Goodwood, Ontario L0C 1A0

International Herbs Co, 31 St Andrews, Toronto, Ontario M5T 1K7

Rosebud Herbs and Produce, RR2, Olds, Alberta T0M 1P0

Forest Glen Herb Farm, County Road 7/1 mile N. County Road 12, Forest, Ontario N0N 1J0

Herb Garden, 94 George Street, Oakville, Ontario L6J 3B7

Stokes Seeds Ltd, 39 James St, St Catherines, Ontario L2R 6R6

Vesey's Seeds Ltd, York RR, PEI C0A 1P0

NEW ZEALAND
Tong Fu Tang, Unit F, 113 Meadowland Drive, Howick, Auckland

Kyber Foods & Spices, 94A Stoddard Rd, Mt Roskill, Auckland

Hingwha Trading Co Ltd, 308-314 Great South Rd, Papatoetoe, Auckland

Davis Trading Co Ltd, 20 Te Puni St, Petone

Mr Chan's, corner Cable & Chafffer Sts, Wellington

Asiana Foods, 77 Tory St, Wellington

Therapeutic Index

Index